RADIOGRAPHY PREP STUDY GUIDE 2024-2025

MASTER THE ARRT RADIOGRAPHY EXAM WITH IN-DEPTH COVERAGE OF PATIENT CARE, SAFETY PROTOCOLS, AND IMAGE PRODUCTION TECHNIQUES | FULL-LENGTH PRACTICE TESTS AND ANSWER EXPLANATIONS

TEST TREASURE PUBLICATION

Test Treasure
PUBLICATION

COPYRIGHT

Email: support@testtreasure.com
Website: www.testtreasure.com

Trademarks

Disclaimer

Governing Law

CONTENTS

INTRODUCTION

Welcome to "Radiography Prep Study Guide 2024-2025" by Test Treasure Publication, your comprehensive companion on the journey to mastering the Radiography Exam. In the dynamic realm of healthcare, where precision and knowledge intersect, this guide is crafted to be your beacon of success.

Understanding the Exam Landscape

Embark on a journey that begins with a detailed overview of the exam's intricacies. Gain insights into the exam pattern, administered body, time frame, and its overarching significance in shaping your radiography career. We pave the way for a nuanced understanding, empowering you to approach the exam with confidence.

Navigating the Sections with Expertise

Dive deep into the core sections, meticulously designed to cover every facet of the Radiography Exam. From the foundational principles of Patient Care to the intricacies of Safety, Image Production, and Procedures, each section is a stepping stone toward mastery. Uncover the nuances of Ethical and Legal Aspects, Principles of Radiation Physics, and more, equipping you with the knowledge essential for success.

Beyond the Textbook: Practical Advice and Strategies

This guide transcends traditional study materials. Beyond the content review, we provide invaluable advice on crafting effective study schedules, planning strategies, and addressing frequently asked questions. Elevate your approach with tested test-taking strategies, arming you with the skills to navigate the exam with finesse.

Practice Tests: A Mirror to Your Preparedness

Put your knowledge to the test with two full-length practice exams, each comprising 100 carefully curated questions. Dive into detailed answer explanations, unraveling the reasoning behind each choice. These practice tests are not just assessments; they are mirrors reflecting your readiness for success.

Additional Resources: Your Gateway to Excellence

Access a curated list of recommended online resources and academic materials, expanding your learning beyond the confines of this guide. Enrich your preparation with external references handpicked to complement your journey toward radiography excellence.

Final Words: Igniting Your Radiography Journey

In the closing chapters, find inspiration and motivation to fuel your journey. Let our final words resonate as a source of encouragement, propelling you toward success in the Radiography Exam and beyond.

Test Treasure Publication invites you to embark on this transformative experience, where learning transcends boundaries, and success becomes a tangible reality. Your radiography future begins here.

OVERVIEW OF THE RADIOGRAPHY EXAM

The Radiography Exam is a pivotal assessment designed to evaluate the competency of aspiring radiologic technologists in the United States. Administered by the American Registry of Radiologic Technologists (ARRT), this comprehensive examination assesses candidates' knowledge and skills across various domains essential for the safe and effective practice of radiography.

Importance of the Radiography Exam:

The significance of the Radiography Exam cannot be overstated, as it serves as a critical benchmark for entry into the field of radiologic technology. Successful completion of this exam is a prerequisite for obtaining licensure and certification, enabling individuals to pursue rewarding careers in medical imaging and radiography.

Key Details:

- **Exam Pattern:** The Radiography Exam typically consists of multiple-choice questions, which assess candidates' understanding of core concepts in radiography.

- **Number of Questions:** The exam comprises a varying number of questions, typically ranging from 100 to 220, covering a comprehensive range of topics.

- **Time Frame:** Candidates are allotted a specified time frame to complete the exam, typically ranging from 3 to 4 hours, depending on the number of questions and the exam format.

- **Scoring:** Each question in the Radiography Exam carries equal weight, with candidates earning points for correct answers and no penalty for incorrect responses. The final score is calculated based on the number of correct responses.

- **Administered by:** The Radiography Exam is administered by the American Registry of Radiologic Technologists (ARRT), a prestigious organization dedicated to promoting excellence in medical imaging and radiation therapy.

Preparation Strategies:

Given the comprehensive nature of the Radiography Exam, thorough preparation is essential for success. Candidates are advised to utilize reputable study guides, practice tests, and review courses to enhance their understanding of key concepts and familiarize themselves with the exam format.

By diligently preparing for the Radiography Exam, aspiring radiologic technologists can embark on their careers with confidence, equipped with the knowledge and skills necessary to provide exceptional patient care and contribute to the field of medical imaging.

Detailed Content Review

Section 1: Patient Care

Ethical and Legal Aspects:

- Explore the ethical foundations of radiography, understanding the legal responsibilities and considerations in patient care.

- Delve into case studies and scenarios, honing your ability to make ethical decisions in a medical context.

Interpersonal Communication:

- Master the art of effective communication with patients, colleagues, and healthcare professionals.

- Practical tips and real-world examples guide you in developing strong interpersonal skills crucial for a successful career in radiography.

Physical Assistance and Monitoring:

- Gain insights into providing physical assistance to patients during imaging procedures.

- Understand the importance of continuous monitoring and ensure patient comfort and safety throughout the radiographic process.

Medical Emergencies:

- Navigate through potential medical emergencies that may arise in a radiography setting.

- Develop a comprehensive understanding of emergency protocols, equipping you to respond confidently and efficiently.

Infection Control:

- Learn the principles of infection control specific to radiography environments.

- Implement best practices to prevent the spread of infections, ensuring a safe and sterile workplace.

Handling and Disposal of Toxic or Hazardous Material:

- Understand the protocols for handling and disposing of toxic or hazardous materials in compliance with safety standards.

- Practical guidelines to ensure environmental sustainability and safety in radiography practice.

Pharmacology:

- Explore the basics of pharmacology relevant to radiography.

- Understand the impact of medications on imaging procedures and patient care.

Section 2: Safety

Principles of Radiation Physics:

- Uncover the fundamental principles governing the physics of radiation in medical imaging.

- Practical applications and scenarios provide a solid foundation for understanding radiation physics.

Biological Aspects of Radiation:

- Delve into the biological effects of radiation on the human body.

- Learn about dose-response relationships and the implications for patient safety.

Minimizing Patient Exposure:

- Explore techniques and strategies to minimize patient exposure to radiation.

- Optimize imaging procedures while prioritizing patient safety and regulatory compliance.

Personnel Protection (ALARA):

- Understand the "As Low As Reasonably Achievable" (ALARA) principle.

- Implement effective measures to protect yourself and colleagues from unnecessary radiation exposure.

Section 3: Image Production

Image Acquisition and Technical Evaluation:

- Master the art of acquiring high-quality radiographic images.

- Develop the skills to critically evaluate technical aspects, ensuring diagnostic excellence.

Equipment Operation and Quality Assurance:

- Gain hands-on knowledge of operating radiographic equipment.

- Implement quality assurance practices to maintain equipment functionality and image quality.

Section 4: Procedures

Head, Spine, and Pelvis Procedures:

- Comprehensive coverage of imaging procedures for the head, spine, and pelvis.

- Detailed step-by-step guides for positioning, technique, and patient communication.

Thorax and Abdomen Procedures:

- In-depth exploration of imaging procedures for the thorax and abdomen.

- Clinical insights and case studies enhance your understanding of diagnostic imaging in these regions.

Extremity Procedures:

- Detailed examination of imaging procedures for the extremities.

- Practical tips for achieving optimal images and ensuring patient comfort.

Practice Tests and Answer Explanations

Two Full-Length Practice Tests:

- Simulate exam conditions with two complete practice tests, each containing 100 questions.

- Evaluate your knowledge across all sections and identify areas for further review.

Detailed Answer Explanations:

- Thorough explanations for each practice test question.

- Understand the reasoning behind correct and incorrect choices, enhancing your learning experience.

Additional Resources and Final Words

Recommended Online Resources and Academic Materials:

- Curated list of external resources to supplement your study journey.

- Access additional materials to broaden your understanding of radiography concepts.

Final Words: Igniting Your Radiography Journey:

- Inspirational closing remarks to motivate and empower you as you embark on your radiography career.

- Find encouragement and confidence to excel in the Radiography Exam and beyond.

STUDY SCHEDULES AND PLANNING ADVICE

Embarking on the journey to conquer the Radiography Exam requires not just knowledge but a strategic approach to study. In this section, we provide comprehensive study schedules and invaluable planning advice to optimize your preparation and ensure success.

Creating Your Study Schedule: A Strategic Blueprint

1. **Assessment of Current Knowledge:**

   - Begin by assessing your current understanding of radiography concepts. Identify strengths and areas that need improvement.

   - Use diagnostic quizzes within the guide to gauge your baseline knowledge and tailor your study plan accordingly.

2. **Sectional Prioritization:**

   - Recognize the weightage of each section in the exam and prioritize your study time accordingly.

   - Allocate more time to sections with higher complexity or where your knowledge may be weaker.

3. **Daily and Weekly Blocks:**

   - Break down your study schedule into daily and weekly blocks.

- Assign specific topics or sections to each block, ensuring comprehensive coverage over time.

4. **Regular Review Sessions:**

- Incorporate regular review sessions to reinforce learned concepts.

- Use flashcards and quick quizzes to keep information fresh in your memory.

5. **Simulated Practice Tests:**

- Integrate simulated practice tests into your schedule, mimicking exam conditions.

- Schedule these tests strategically to monitor your progress and identify areas for improvement.

Planning Advice for Effective Preparation

1. **Consistency over Cramming:**

- Aim for consistent, daily study sessions rather than last-minute cramming.

- Spacing out your study sessions enhances long-term retention and understanding.

2. **Active Learning Techniques:**

- Engage in active learning by teaching concepts to yourself or others.

- Use mnemonic devices, mind maps, and visualization techniques to reinforce key points.

3. **Balanced Study Approach:**

- Ensure a balanced approach to studying all sections.

- Rotate between different topics to maintain interest and prevent burnout.

4. **Utilization of Resources:**

- Leverage the additional resources provided, including recommended online materials.

- Expand your understanding with diverse resources that complement the guide.

5. **Adaptability in Planning:**

- Stay flexible in your study plan to adapt to unexpected challenges or opportunities.

- Adjust your schedule based on progress and identified areas of focus.

6. **Self-Care and Well-being:**

- Prioritize self-care and well-being throughout your study journey.

- Ensure adequate breaks, sleep, and relaxation to maintain a healthy study-life balance.

7. **Motivational Checkpoints:**

- Set achievable milestones and celebrate your successes along the way.

- Use motivational checkpoints to keep yourself inspired and focused on the ultimate goal.

With this strategic study schedule and planning advice, you're not just preparing for an exam; you're cultivating a deep understanding of radiography principles that will serve you well in your future career.

FREQUENTLY ASKED QUESTIONS

Q1: How is this study guide different from other resources available?

A1: Our study guide goes beyond traditional exam preparation. It acts as your mentor, providing a holistic approach to radiography. From comprehensive content reviews to practical advice, we focus on building not just exam competence but a solid foundation for your future career.

Q2: How should I use the diagnostic quizzes within the guide?

A2: The diagnostic quizzes are designed to help you assess your baseline knowledge. Take these quizzes at the beginning of your preparation to identify strengths and weaknesses. Tailor your study plan based on the results to make your preparation targeted and efficient.

Q3: Can I solely rely on this guide for exam preparation?

A3: While the guide is a robust resource, we recommend supplementing your study with the additional resources provided. These include recommended online materials and academic references, offering a well-rounded understanding of radiography concepts.

Q4: How should I approach the two full-length practice tests?

A4: Treat the practice tests as simulated exam experiences. Allocate dedicated time, create a quiet environment, and adhere to the time constraints. After completing each test, thoroughly review the detailed answer explanations to understand your performance and areas that need improvement.

Q5: How can I stay motivated throughout my study journey?

A5: Setting achievable milestones, celebrating small victories, and incorporating motivational checkpoints into your study plan can help you stay motivated. Remember the bigger picture—each step brings you closer to success in the Radiography Exam and your future career.

Q6: Is there a recommended order for studying the sections?

A6: While the guide provides a suggested order, feel free to adapt based on your preferences. If you find certain sections more challenging, consider addressing them earlier in your study plan. The key is to maintain a balanced approach and ensure coverage of all sections.

Q7: How can I make the most of the recommended online resources?

A7: Explore the recommended online resources to deepen your understanding. Use them to explore specific topics, access additional practice questions, or gain insights from different perspectives. Diversifying your sources enhances the richness of your preparation.

Q8: Can I reach out for additional support or clarification?

A8: Absolutely! If you encounter challenges or have questions during your preparation, don't hesitate to seek support. Utilize forums, online communities, or reach out to fellow students. Additionally, stay tuned for updates on our website for any clarifications or additional resources.

Remember, your success in the Radiography Exam is not just about passing a test; it's about building a foundation for a successful career. Embrace the journey, stay focused, and use this guide as your compass to navigate the path to excellence.

Section 1: Patient Care

Ethical and Legal Aspects

Patient rights form the foundation of ethical practice in radiography. Every individual seeking healthcare is entitled to certain fundamental rights, and it is the duty of the radiographer to respect and protect these rights. As we delve into this topic, we shall examine the key patient rights that radiographers must uphold.

Confidentiality is one such right. Patients must be assured that their personal and medical information will remain strictly confidential. This ethical principle emphasizes the importance of trust between the patient and the radiographer. By maintaining confidentiality, radiographers not only preserve the privacy of their patients but also create an environment where individuals feel safe to share sensitive information. As guardians of confidential patient data, radiographers must adhere to legal regulations such as the Health Insurance Portability and Accountability Act (HIPAA) and ensure that patient records are accessed only by authorized personnel.

In addition to confidentiality, the principle of informed consent upholds the autonomy of patients. Through informed consent, patients have the right to be fully informed about their diagnostic procedures, including potential risks and benefits. Radiographers must engage in open and honest communication, presenting information in a manner that patients can understand. This lays the groundwork for shared decision-making and enables patients to actively participate in their healthcare journey.

Professional codes of conduct further outline the ethical standards that radiographers must follow. These codes provide explicit guidelines on issues such as honesty, integrity, and professional competence. By adhering to these codes, radiographers ensure that their practice aligns with the highest ethical standards. They prioritize the best interests of their patients, always placing their needs above all others.

Apart from ethical considerations, radiographers must also be well-versed in the legal obligations that govern their practice. Understanding the laws and regulations that pertain to the field of radiography is essential for providing safe and effective care.

Radiographers must be aware of the legal requirements surrounding the protection of patient health information. Breaches in confidentiality can have serious consequences, resulting in legal consequences for both the individual radiographer and the healthcare facility they work for. It is their duty to safeguard patient information and to report any breach or unauthorized access promptly.

Additionally, radiographers must familiarize themselves with the laws related to professional liability. In the course of their work, they may encounter situations where their actions or decisions have direct implications for patient well-being. Understanding the legal framework surrounding professional liability empowers radiographers with the knowledge needed to navigate potential challenges and protect both themselves and their patients.

In conclusion, exploring the ethical principles and legal obligations in the field of radiography is imperative for radiographers to provide exemplary care. By upholding patient rights, maintaining confidentiality, and adhering to professional codes of conduct, radiographers contribute to a compassionate and ethical healthcare setting. Similarly, remaining knowledgeable about the legal framework within which they operate helps radiographers fulfill their responsibilities and mitigate potential legal risks. Ultimately, the dedication to ethical and legal aspects ensures that radiographers maintain the highest standards of professional practice, inspiring confidence and trust in their patients.

Interpersonal Communication

In the field of radiography, effective communication is not only crucial for obtaining accurate medical history but also for establishing a bond of trust and empathy with patients. As healthcare professionals, we must recognize that communication is not limited to verbal interactions alone. It encompasses a range of skills and techniques that allow us to connect with patients on a deeper level, alleviating their fears and concerns while ensuring their well-being remains at the forefront of our practice.

Active Listening: The Art of Hearing Beyond Words

Active listening forms the bedrock of effective communication. It goes beyond simply hearing the words a patient utters and delves into understanding the emotions behind them. To truly engage in active listening, one must create a safe and inviting environment where patients feel comfortable expressing their thoughts and concerns openly. As a radiographer, I strive to establish a genuine connection with every patient, making eye contact, maintaining an open posture, and offering words of reassurance to let them know they have been heard. This technique not only helps me gather crucial information about their condition but also empowers patients, as they feel valued and respected throughout the interaction.

Empathy: The Bridge to Human Connection

Empathy is the cornerstone of interpersonal communication in healthcare. It allows us to step into the shoes of our patients, understanding their fears, anxieties, and hopes. By acknowledging and validating their emotions, we can create a compassionate and supportive environment that instills a sense of trust within patients. I often find myself taking a moment to empathize with the challenges they may be facing, whether it's a fear of the unknown or the vulnerability that comes with being unwell. By expressing empathy through my words, tone, and body language, I aim to foster a sense of understanding and camaraderie, helping patients feel heard, seen, and cared for during their journey.

Non-Verbal Communication: The Unspoken Language of Comfort

While verbal communication is undoubtedly important, we must not underestimate the power of non-verbal cues in building rapport. Our body language, facial expressions, and gestures can communicate empathy, compassion, and reassurance without uttering a single word. As a radiographer, I am conscious of the messages my non-verbal cues convey to patients. I maintain an open and friendly demeanor, mirroring their emotions to show solidarity and convey a sense of understanding. Offering a gentle touch on their shoulder or maintaining a warm smile can go a long way in establishing trust and creating a comfortable environment for patients.

Conclusion: Cultivating Meaningful Connections

Examining effective communication techniques for building rapport with patients highlights the significance of establishing a connection that transcends the boundaries of a clinical setting. Active listening, empathy, and non-verbal communication all contribute to building trust, assuaging fears, and fostering a healing environment. By incorporating these techniques into our daily practice, radiographers can create a safe space where patients feel valued, understood, and supported. It is in these moments of connection that we truly fulfill our role as compassionate healthcare professionals, guiding patients on their journey to recovery and affirming our commitment to their well-being.

Physical Assistance and Monitoring

When it comes to assisting patients with transfers and positioning, it is essential to prioritize their safety above all else. Test Treasure Publication offers detailed instructions on the correct techniques to lift, support, and move patients with varying levels of mobility. We emphasize the significance of maintaining proper body mechanics to prevent injury to yourself and the patient. By mastering these techniques, you can ensure a smooth and secure transfer experience for both parties involved.

Moreover, our study materials enlighten you about the significance of monitoring vital signs during patient assistance. Vital signs serve as indicators of a patient's overall well-being and offer valuable insights into their physiological condition. We provide a comprehensive breakdown of the vital signs that radiographers should monitor, including heart rate, blood pressure, respiration rate, and temperature. By meticulously observing these vital signs, you can identify any abnormalities or distress that may arise during physical activities.

Recognizing signs of distress is an essential skill that every radiographer must possess. Our comprehensive study guide equips you with the knowledge to identify and respond to distress signals promptly. We delve into the common signs of distress, such as rapid breathing, sweating, and pallor, helping you develop the observational skills necessary to identify these indicators in real-life scenarios. By mastering the art of recognizing distress, you can respond swiftly and effectively, alleviating any potential harm or discomfort to your patients.

At Test Treasure Publication, we recognize that physical assistance and monitoring arc integral components of providing quality care to patients in the field of radiography. Our study materials go beyond theoretical knowledge, incorporating real-life scenarios and practical tips to ensure a seamless and patient-centered approach to physical assistance. With our guidance, you will gain the confidence to navigate any situation that requires physical assistance, while also honing your ability to monitor vital signs and recognize distress signals.

In conclusion, the chapter on Physical Assistance and Monitoring in the Radiography Prep Study Guide 2024-2025 from Test Treasure Publication provides a comprehensive understanding of the necessary skills and techniques to safely assist patients in transfers and positioning. By emphasizing the significance of monitoring vital signs and recognizing signs of distress, we strive to equip radiographers with the knowledge and confidence to provide exceptional care. Join us at Test Treasure Publication, and together, let us journey toward extraordinary success in your radiography career.

Medical Emergencies

In an emergency scenario, every second counts. Therefore, it is imperative that you familiarize yourself with basic life support techniques to provide immediate care to patients in distress. Cardiovascular emergencies, such as cardiac arrest or myocardial infarction, require prompt intervention to maximize chances of survival. This guide will take you through the step-by-step process of performing cardiopulmonary resuscitation (CPR) and using automated external defibrillators (AEDs) effectively.

Another critical aspect of preparing for medical emergencies is understanding and following emergency protocols. It is crucial to be familiar with the emergency response plan of the healthcare facility in which you work. This includes knowing the location of emergency equipment, such as crash carts and emergency medications, as well as the emergency contact numbers and codes specific to your workplace. Additionally, being aware of the chain of command and communication channels during emergencies will ensure a well-coordinated response.

Test Treasure Publication takes a comprehensive approach to teaching emergency preparedness, emphasizing not only the technical skills but also the importance of remaining calm and composed under pressure. We delve into the psychological aspects of emergency situations, discussing strategies to maintain a clear mind and make effective decisions in high-stress environments. Our study materials include realistic case studies and simulations that allow you to practice your emergency response skills in a controlled setting, ensuring preparedness for real-life emergencies.

Furthermore, we recognize the significance of collaboration and teamwork in effectively managing medical emergencies. In radiography, you are part of a multidisciplinary team comprising radiologists, nurses, and other healthcare professionals. Understanding each team member's role in an emergency and effectively communicating and coordinating with them are vital for successful outcomes. Test Treasure Publication fosters this collaborative spirit through interactive exercises and scenarios that promote teamwork and effective communication skills.

To ensure that you are up-to-date with the latest advancements and protocols in emergency medicine, we constantly update our study materials to reflect the most current guidelines. Our team of expert educators and healthcare professionals work diligently to provide you with accurate and reliable information, empowering you to excel in your radiography practice.

In conclusion, preparing radiographers to respond swiftly and appropriately in medical emergencies is a fundamental aspect of our study guide. With a strong focus on basic life support techniques and emergency protocols, we aim to equip you with the skills and knowledge needed to confidently handle any emergency situation. Test Treasure Publication is committed to your success and safety, guiding you on this extraordinary journey of becoming a skilled and compassionate radiographer who is prepared to face any challenge that may arise.

Infection Control

Welcome to the chapter on infection control, an indispensable component of radiography that encompasses an array of practices aimed at safeguarding patients, healthcare professionals, and the surrounding environment from harmful microorganisms. In this section, we will delve into the paramountcy of infection control in radiography and expound upon the key strategies employed to mitigate the risk of healthcare-associated infections.

In the realm of radiography, infection control assumes a paramount importance. The delicate nature of the medical field necessitates an unwavering commitment to maintaining strict infection control protocols. As a radiographer, you will find yourself at the forefront of patient care, regularly interacting with individuals who may be immunocompromised or vulnerable to infections. It is your duty to prioritize their well-being and ensure that radiography procedures are carried out under the safest possible circumstances.

Hand hygiene serves as the cornerstone of effective infection control. By adhering to stringent hand hygiene practices, radiographers can significantly reduce the transmission of microorganisms from their hands to patients and vice versa. Regular handwashing with soap and water, or alternatively, the use of alcohol-based hand sanitizers, is imperative before and after every interaction with patients or contaminated surfaces. Scrubbing hands for at least 20 seconds, focusing on all surfaces, including the back of hands, between fingers, and under nails, is vital for complete decontamination.

Personal protective equipment (PPE) is another crucial aspect of infection control in radiography. It serves as a barrier between you and potentially infectious materials, minimizing the risk of exposure. At Test Treasure Publication, we emphasize the significance of donning appropriate PPE before entering any patient's room or performing radiography procedures. This may include wearing gloves, masks, gowns, and protective eyewear, depending on the nature of the procedure and potential hazards involved. Additionally, proper disposal of PPE is paramount to prevent cross-contamination and ensure a safe and clean environment.

Infection control in radiography also encompasses proper disinfection techniques. Disinfection protocols should be meticulously followed to eradicate microorganisms, preventing their proliferation and transmission. It is essential to use appropriate disinfectants, following the manufacturer's instructions, for surfaces, equipment, and accessories used during radiography procedures. Paying close attention to frequently touched surfaces, such as X-ray machines, table surfaces, and control panels, significantly reduces the risk of contamination. Your dedication to thorough disinfection practices will contribute to the overall reduction of healthcare-associated infections, ensuring optimal patient care.

To further enhance infection control in radiography, we at Test Treasure Publication recommend the following strategies:

1. Consistent and regular training: Stay up-to-date with the latest infection control guidelines, trends, and research. Attend seminars, webinars, and conferences that focus on infection control practices specific to radiography. Engage in continuous education to deepen your understanding and mastery of infection control protocols.

2. Collaborative approach: Foster a culture of infection control within your workplace. Encourage open communication, collaboration, and accountability among radiographers, healthcare professionals, and support staff. Everyone should be actively involved in upholding infection control standards and proactively identifying opportunities for improvement.

3. Thoughtful patient education: Empower patients with knowledge and awareness about infection control practices. Clearly explain the steps you take to ensure their safety throughout the radiography process. Encourage them to ask questions and address any concerns they may have. Educating patients as active participants in their own care helps foster a sense of shared responsibility.

4. Monitoring and assessment: Regularly evaluate the effectiveness of infection control practices in your radiography department. Implement robust monitoring processes to identify potential areas for improvement. This may include observations, audits, and feedback from patients and colleagues. By actively seeking feedback and monitoring infection control measures, you can continuously enhance the safety of your radiography practice.

In conclusion, infection control is of paramount importance in radiography. It requires a steadfast commitment to hand hygiene, proper utilization of personal protective equipment, and adherence to disinfection protocols. By meticulously following these practices and implementing additional strategies, we can collectively ensure the safety and well-being of patients and healthcare professionals alike. At Test Treasure Publication, we are dedicated to equipping and empowering aspiring radiographers with the knowledge and skills needed to excel in their profession, including advocating for comprehensive infection control. Together, we can minimize the risk of healthcare-associated infections and build a safer future for radiography.

Handling and Disposal of Toxic or Hazardous Material

When it comes to handling toxic or hazardous materials, there is no room for complacency or negligence. The repercussions of mishandling such substances can be severe, both in terms of immediate danger and long-term health effects. Thus, our study guide places a strong emphasis on the importance of following established protocols and regulatory requirements. By adhering to these guidelines, radiography professionals can ensure the safety of themselves, their colleagues, and the environment.

To provide an in-depth understanding, we delve into various types of toxic or hazardous materials encountered in radiography. From radiocontrast agents to biohazardous waste, we explore the unique characteristics and risks associated with each substance. By comprehending the inherent hazards, radiographers can make informed decisions when it comes to handling and storage.

In addition to outlining these risks, our study guide goes one step further by equipping students with the knowledge of appropriate handling techniques. We provide detailed instructions on the use of personal protective equipment, such as gloves, goggles, and respirators, to minimize exposure to potentially harmful substances. Moreover, we emphasize the significance of proper labeling and containment to prevent accidental spills or leakages.

The safe storage of toxic or hazardous materials is another crucial aspect that our study guide addresses. We highlight the importance of storing substances in designated areas, away from incompatible materials and potential sources of ignition. By organizing storage spaces systematically and implementing stringent inventory management, radiography professionals can ensure a safe working environment and swift response in case of emergencies.

Equally significant is the proper disposal of toxic or hazardous materials. Our study guide stresses the adherence to local, state, and federal regulations governing the disposal of such substances. We provide a comprehensive breakdown of different disposal methods, ranging from segregation and treatment to incineration and burial. By familiarizing themselves with these protocols, radiography practitioners can contribute to the preservation of both human health and the environment.

Throughout this chapter, Test Treasure Publication incorporates real-life case studies and scenarios to enhance the learning experience. By presenting students with practical challenges and dilemmas, we encourage critical thinking and decision-making skills. By grappling with these complex situations in a safe learning environment, radiography professionals will be better prepared to handle real-world issues.

In conclusion, the handling and disposal of toxic or hazardous materials is a critical aspect of radiography practice. At Test Treasure Publication, we are committed to equipping students with the knowledge and skills necessary to navigate this challenging terrain. By providing comprehensive guidelines, emphasizing the importance of established protocols, and inspiring a deep sense of responsibility, we empower radiography professionals to ensure safety, protect their patients, and contribute to the advancement of the field.

Pharmacology

In this section, we will embark on an enlightening journey, exploring the intricacies of pharmacology relevant to radiography. Together, we will unravel the mystery behind the common medications used in imaging procedures, their indications, contraindications, and potential side effects. We understand the importance of equipping you with a comprehensive understanding of these essential drugs to guide you in your role as a radiographer.

Medications play a pivotal role in various imaging procedures, aiding in the diagnosis, management, and treatment of diverse medical conditions. Therefore, it is imperative to be well-versed in the pharmacological agents used in radiography. By familiarizing yourself with these medications, you will not only be able to administer them safely but also comprehend their impact on imaging outcomes.

Throughout this section, we will meticulously explore the different categories of medications commonly employed in radiography, each with its unique function and purpose. From iodinated contrast agents to sedatives and analgesics, we will delve into the depths of their mechanisms, indications, and contraindications.

Furthermore, we will shine a light on the potential side effects that may arise from medication administration during imaging procedures. Our comprehensive discussion will empower you to recognize and manage these side effects, ensuring the utmost safety and well-being of your patients.

Above all, we emphasize the importance of medication safety and administration. At Test Treasure Publication, we understand the critical role you play as a radiographer in the healthcare team, ensuring that medications are administered accurately and in accordance with established protocols. We will guide you through best practices in medication safety, equipping you with the tools and knowledge necessary to mitigate risks and prioritize patient well-being.

In summary, this section on pharmacology is designed to immerse you in the intricacies of medications relevant to radiography. It is our goal to empower you with a profound understanding of these drugs, enabling you to provide exceptional patient care while upholding the highest standards of medication safety. Together, let us navigate this chapter, illuminating the path to mastery in pharmacology for radiography.

SECTION 2: SAFETY

Principles of Radiation Physics

Firstly, we embark on a journey to understand the nature of radiation itself. What is it that sets radiation apart from other forms of energy? How does it come to be? These questions drive our exploration of the structure and behavior of radiation at its core. Through meticulous research and analysis, we provide you with a comprehensive understanding of this elusive phenomenon.

Once grasping the nature of radiation, we dive into the vast ocean of its properties. From the ethereal waves of gamma rays to the energetic streams of x-rays, we unravel the electromagnetic spectrum, painting a vivid picture of the diverse forms radiation can take. With expertly curated visuals and detailed explanations, we illuminate the intricacies that make each type of radiation unique and valuable in various applications.

Building upon this foundation, we then dive into the vital concept of ionizing radiation. By exploring the mechanisms that enable radiation to ionize atoms and molecules, we equip you with a profound understanding of the potential dangers and benefits associated with this remarkable force. Immersed in an array of case studies and real-world examples, you will witness the far-reaching implications that ionizing radiation has on medicine, industry, and the environment.

With the foundations laid firmly, we set out to tackle the complex matter of radiation units of measurement. In this section, we guide you through the intricacies of the Roentgen, Rad, Rem, and other significant measurement units. By delving into their origins, definitions, and conversion factors, we provide you with the tools necessary to navigate the complex web of radiation measurement with confidence and accuracy.

Throughout this journey, we remain steadfast in our commitment to your success. Our study materials serve as your trusted mentor, enriching your learning experience and inspiring you to excel. We pride ourselves on our impeccable attention to detail, ensuring that each concept is meticulously explained, enabling you to grasp even the most intricate intricacies.

Radiation physics is a subject that lies at the heart of radiography. Hence, understanding its principles is an essential step towards becoming a proficient and knowledgeable radiographer. With our study guide in hand, we invite you to embark on a transformative journey, where ordinary learning transcends into a profound understanding of the principles that govern the world of radiation physics. Let us empower you to take on the challenges that lie ahead and illuminate the path to extraordinary success.

Biological Aspects of Radiation

As we embark on this intellectual expedition, it is imperative that we first understand the fundamental notion of radiation and its impact on biological systems. Radiation, although a powerful tool in the fields of medicine and industry, can have profound effects on living organisms when not managed with utmost care.

Our voyage begins with an exploration into the acute effects of radiation exposure. This term refers to the immediate and severe consequences resulting from high-dosage radiation, often encountered during a nuclear accident or a nuclear weapon detonation. The magnitude of these effects can be devastating, wreaking havoc on the exposed individual's genetic material, leading to radiation sickness, organ failure, and even death.

However, the impact of radiation on living organisms is not limited to acute effects only. The consequences of long-term or repeated radiation exposure, known as chronic effects, warrant our careful consideration. Chronic effects, while less immediately apparent, are equally significant in their potential long-term impact. They can manifest in various forms, such as an increased risk of developing cancer, genetic mutations, and even hereditary defects in future generations.

To better comprehend the intricate relationship between radiation exposure and its biological effects, let us explore the concept of radiation dose-response relationships. This notion seeks to establish a correlation between the intensity or dose of radiation received and the resulting biological response. By scrutinizing this relationship, scientists have been able to ascertain that as radiation dosage escalates, the risk of adverse effects also increases proportionately.

Nonetheless, the story does not end here. Within the realm of radiation's biological effects, lie two critical categories: stochastic and deterministic effects. Stochastic effects refer to those effects that occur randomly and become more likely with increased radiation exposure. These effects are dose-dependent, meaning that the probability of occurrence escalates with higher levels of radiation exposure. Examples of stochastic effects include cancer development and the risk of genetic mutations.

On the other hand, deterministic effects exhibit a different set of characteristics. Deterministic effects, unlike stochastic effects, have a threshold below which they do not occur. However, once this threshold is surpassed, the severity of the effect increases with the dosage of radiation. Some examples of deterministic effects include skin burns, organ failure, and cataracts.

Through our voyage into the biological aspects of radiation, we have discovered the intricacies of radiation's impact on living organisms. From the immediate wrath of acute effects to the insidious and long-term consequences of chronic effects, the ramifications of radiation exposure have far-reaching implications. By understanding the dose-response relationship, we gain insights into the direct correlation between the intensity of radiation and its biological repercussions. Furthermore, the classification of stochastic and deterministic effects reveals the unique nature of each category, adding depth to our understanding of radiation's biological impact.

As I conclude this chapter, I invite you, dear readers, to reflect upon the fragile balance between harnessing the power of radiation for medical and industrial advancements while safeguarding the well-being of living organisms. The study of biological aspects of radiation serves as a reminder of the responsibility we bear as guardians of this knowledge. Let us embark on this journey with a deep sense of awe and reverence, knowing that through understanding and vigilance, we can ensure a future of boundless opportunities for generations to come.

Until next time, fellow learners, I bid you farewell and bestow upon you the wisdom gained in our exploration of the biological aspects of radiation. May this knowledge guide you on your path to extraordinary success in your radiography pursuits.

Minimizing Patient Exposure

At the heart of minimizing patient exposure lies the concept of optimization principles. These principles guide healthcare professionals in achieving the delicate balance between acquiring high-quality diagnostic images and limiting the radiation dose received by patients. Through a thorough understanding of these principles, radiographers can customize imaging protocols to suit the individual needs of each patient, tailoring the imaging technique and radiation dose to specific clinical indications.

In addition to optimization principles, healthcare professionals can utilize a range of dose reduction methods to further minimize patient exposure. One such method is the use of automatic exposure control (AEC) devices, which adjust the radiation dose based on the patient's anatomy and the desired image quality. By allowing for precise dose modulation, AEC devices ensure that the appropriate amount of radiation is delivered, minimizing unnecessary exposure.

Furthermore, the use of shielding devices is an essential aspect of minimizing patient exposure. Lead aprons, thyroid collars, and other specialized shields act as barriers, effectively blocking radiation from reaching sensitive areas of the patient's body. By strategically positioning these shielding devices, radiographers can safeguard vital organs, such as the reproductive organs and thyroid gland, from unnecessary radiation exposure.

To effectively implement these strategies and techniques, healthcare professionals must stay abreast of the latest research and technological advancements in radiography. Continuous education and professional development programs help radiographers enhance their knowledge and skills, enabling them to provide the highest standard of care while minimizing patient exposure.

Test Treasure Publication recognizes the significance of equipping aspiring radiographers with this in-depth understanding of patient exposure minimization. Our study materials not only cover the theoretical foundations but also provide practical scenarios and case studies to deepen comprehension. By immersing students in a comprehensive learning experience, we empower them to make informed decisions and take the necessary steps to ensure patient safety.

In conclusion, the responsibility of minimizing patient exposure to radiation during imaging procedures rests squarely on the shoulders of healthcare professionals. With optimization principles, dose reduction methods, and the use of shielding devices as their arsenal, radiographers can deliver the highest-quality care while safeguarding patients from unnecessary radiation exposure. At Test Treasure Publication, we strive to provide a comprehensive study guide that educates and inspires future radiographers, preparing them to prioritize patient safety and access the path to extraordinary success.

Personnel Protection (ALARA)

One of the fundamental principles that underpin personnel protection in radiography is the ALARA principle, which stands for "As Low As Reasonably Achievable." This principle guides us to minimize radiation doses and risks to workers, patients, and the general public while still achieving the necessary diagnostic information. ALARA serves as our guiding light, reminding us that unnecessary radiation exposure poses potentially grave risks to health and well-being.

To ensure the effective implementation of the ALARA principle, regular radiation monitoring is essential. In the world of radiography, it is of paramount importance to consistently measure and record radiation exposure levels. This allows us to identify potential areas of concern and take appropriate action to minimize radiation doses. By keeping a close eye on these levels, we can swiftly detect any anomalies and intervene as necessary, thereby safeguarding the health and safety of everyone involved.

Yet, as crucial as radiation monitoring is, it is equally vital to equip individuals with personal protective equipment (PPE). These specialized garments and accessories effectively shield practitioners from unnecessary radiation exposure. From lead aprons and thyroid shields to goggles and gloves, this armor provides a tangible barrier between the human body and harmful radiation. At Test Treasure

Publication, we understand the significance of investing in premium quality PPE, as sub-par equipment could undermine the protection it is designed to offer.

However, protection extends beyond just the physical realm. It requires a holistic approach that encompasses safe work practices. To minimize radiation exposure, it is imperative to follow strict protocols and established procedures. This involves maintaining a safe distance from the radiation source, using appropriate shielding techniques, and ensuring proper ventilation in radiography rooms. Moreover, we advocate for the innovative use of technologies such as remote-controlled devices and shielding materials to further mitigate occupational risks.

At Test Treasure Publication, we understand that exceptional education is not merely about achieving high scores on exams. It is about fostering a culture of safety and well-being among practitioners. Our study materials provide comprehensive guidance on all facets of radiography, including the vital need for personnel protection. We help learners develop an in-depth understanding of the ALARA principle, radiation monitoring techniques, the proper use of personal protective equipment, and the implementation of safe work practices.

In this endeavor, we are committed to going beyond traditional learning methods. Our study guides serve as mentors, empowering students to take charge of their own safety and that of their colleagues. By cultivating a community-driven approach, we encourage the sharing of knowledge, experiences, and best practices among aspiring radiographers. Test Treasure Publication isn't just a publisher—it is our ethical responsibility to ensure that we equip future radiography professionals with the knowledge and skills they need to excel in their careers while safeguarding their own well-being.

As we continue this journey together, let us remember that personnel protection in radiography is not just a box to be ticked—it is a matter of utmost significance. By applying the principles of ALARA, embracing radiation monitoring, utilizing personal protective equipment effectively, and adhering to safe work practices, we can create a safer and healthier environment for all radiography professionals. Let Test Treasure Publication be your trusted guide as we pave the way toward extraordinary success and a future that is filled with boundless opportunities.

SECTION 3: IMAGE PRODUCTION

Image Acquisition and Technical Evaluation

To begin, let us explore the fundamentals of image acquisition. Our comprehensive overview covers the essential components of positioning, exposure factors, and image receptor selection. Positioned as guardians of optimal imaging, radiographers must possess a deep understanding of anatomical landmarks and optimal patient positioning. Mastery of this art enables us to obtain the best possible image, minimizing artifacts and maximizing diagnostic yield.

The second critical aspect of image acquisition is the mastery of exposure factors. As radiographers, we must consider the interplay of kilovolt peak (kVp), milliamperes (mA), exposure time, and source-image distance (SID) to strike the perfect balance between image quality and patient radiation dose. With precision and finesse, we manipulate these variables to capture images that showcase the intricate details of the human body.

Lastly, we explore the significance of image receptor selection. Whether it is the classic film-screen combination or the burgeoning digital radiography, radiographers navigate the ever-evolving landscape of technology to select the most appropriate receptors. We empower ourselves with knowledge, evaluating the pros and cons of each modality to achieve unparalleled clarity and definition in our images.

But our responsibility does not end at image acquisition. The images we capture undergo meticulous technical evaluation to ensure diagnostic quality. As radiographers, we are both artists and scientists, trained to dissect the smallest nuances within an image. We scrutinize each image, assessing factors such as density, contrast, and sharpness to ensure the diagnostic accuracy demanded by healthcare professionals.

Yet, our role in image interpretation does not stop at the technical evaluation. By virtue of our expertise, we become essential collaborators in the diagnostic process. Radiographers possess a unique perspective, having witnessed the full journey from image acquisition to interpretation. We become the bridge, conveying our observations and insights to the interpreting radiologist, ensuring seamless and accurate diagnosis.

In conclusion, image acquisition and technical evaluation go hand in hand, each complementing the other in the quest for precise and impactful radiographic imaging. At Test Treasure Publication, we recognize the criticality of this skill set and have designed this study guide to empower you with the knowledge and understanding necessary to excel in this dynamic field. With our comprehensive resources and unwavering commitment to your success, we invite you to embark on this enlightening journey, transforming yourself into a radiographer who not only captures images but shapes the future of healthcare through impeccable image acquisition and technical evaluation.

Equipment Operation and Quality Assurance

At the heart of radiography lies the X-ray generator, a powerful apparatus that produces the necessary X-rays for capturing images. Understanding its operation is paramount to ensuring accurate and high-quality radiographic examinations. This chapter will demystify the mechanisms behind X-ray generation, shedding light on concepts such as thermionic emission, tube current, and tube voltage.

Our in-depth exploration of X-ray generators will empower you with the knowledge to manipulate these variables effectively, enabling precise control of image quality.

In the ever-evolving landscape of radiography, digital imaging systems have emerged as a revolutionary advancement. Gone are the days of film-based radiography, as digital technology now dominates the field. Through this chapter, you will gain a comprehensive understanding of digital image acquisition, processing, and display systems. Dive into the world of direct and indirect digital radiography, familiarizing yourself with different types of image receptors, such as amorphous silicon, amorphous selenium, and charge-coupled devices. Delve into the intricacies of pixel size, bit depth, and spatial resolution, all of which significantly impact the radiographic image.

While the prowess of X-ray generators and digital imaging systems cannot be understated, maintaining their optimal performance is a critical aspect of radiographic practice. Quality assurance programs play a vital role in ensuring that equipment functions optimally and consistently produces accurate images. Throughout this chapter, you will discover the importance of regular equipment calibration, image receptor checks, and detector cleaning. By understanding quality assurance procedures, you will be equipped to detect and address potential issues before they compromise the integrity of radiographic examinations.

Of course, even the most diligently maintained equipment can encounter technical issues from time to time. Troubleshooting common problems is a skill every radiographer should possess. This chapter will guide you through troubleshooting procedures, equipping you with the ability to identify and resolve common technical issues efficiently. From diagnosing faulty tubes and cables to addressing image artifacts, you will develop the expertise to navigate through challenges with ease.

As we embark on this quest to unravel the secrets of equipment operation and quality assurance in radiography, I invite you to immerse yourself in the captivating world of X-ray generators, image intensifiers, and digital imaging systems. Together, let us embark on a journey that will empower you and illuminate the path to extraordinary success in your radiographic endeavors.

Section 4: Procedures

Head, Spine, and Pelvis Procedures

Radiographic imaging of the head, spine, and pelvis requires a meticulous approach, harnessing the power of positioning techniques, exposure factors, and anatomical considerations. Each procedure holds its own unique challenges, necessitating a careful balance between technical precision and patient comfort.

Let us first venture into the realm of head imaging, where the intricate structures of the skull and brain come to life on the radiographic canvas. When it comes to capturing images of the cranium, it is crucial to employ positioning techniques that provide the utmost clarity and diagnostic value. This involves meticulous alignment of the patient's head, ensuring that the skull is parallel to the image receptor and that the mid-sagittal plane is accurately positioned. Exposure factors play a crucial role in obtaining the finest details while minimizing radiation dose. Careful consideration must also be given to anatomical variations, such as the presence of dental hardware or cranial pathology, which may require modified positioning techniques.

Next, we step into the captivating realm of spinal imaging, where the delicate interplay between bone and soft tissue comes into focus. Radiographic procedures involving the spine require a nuanced understanding of the complex vertebral column, as well as positioning techniques that effectively capture the desired anatomical region. Patient cooperation is key in achieving accurate spinal images, necessitating proper communication and reassurance. Exposure factors must be carefully selected to optimize image quality while minimizing radiation dosage. Anatomical considerations, such as the presence of scoliosis or spinal implants, require a tailored approach to positioning and image acquisition.

Finally, we venture into the realm of pelvis imaging, where the intricate bony structures and visceral organs merge in a tapestry of complexity. Radiographic procedures involving the pelvis demand a thorough understanding of pelvic anatomy and a keen eye for positioning techniques that capture the area of interest. Alignment of the patient's pelvis to the image receptor is crucial to ensure accurate representation of the bony landmarks and soft tissue structures. Exposure factors, once again, need to be chosen judiciously, considering the presence of pelvic pathology such as fractures or congenital abnormalities. Anatomical considerations, such as the variations in pelvic alignment and body habitus, may require tailored positioning techniques to obtain diagnostically meaningful images.

As we come to the end of this chapter on head, spine, and pelvis procedures, we emerge with a newfound appreciation for the intricate dance between technology, anatomy, and patient care. The art of attaining high-quality radiographic images in these areas relies on a deep understanding of positioning techniques, exposure factors, and anatomical considerations. It is with this knowledge that radiologic technologists can unveil the hidden secrets within the head, spine, and pelvis, leaving no stone unturned in their pursuit of accurate diagnosis and patient care.

Thorax and Abdomen Procedures

Positioning is key in obtaining accurate and diagnostic images of the thorax and abdomen. We delve deep into the intricacies of every position, meticulously guiding students through the process step by step. From the basic posteroanterior (PA) and anteroposterior (AP) chest projections to the more specialized views like the lordotic position and lateral decubitus, we leave no stone unturned. Our study materials provide clear illustrations and detailed explanations, ensuring that students grasp the nuances of each position and enhance their proficiency.

But positioning is not the sole aspect to consider. Exposure factors also play a vital role in obtaining high-quality radiographic images. Our study guide equips students with the knowledge of how to select appropriate exposure factors for thorax and abdomen procedures, including factors like kilovoltage (kV), milliampere-seconds (mAs), and source-to-image distance (SID). We dive into the theoretical foundations, explaining the science behind exposure factors and their impact on the image quality. By understanding and applying these factors accurately, students will be able to produce images that meet diagnostic standards.

While the technical aspects of radiographic procedures are essential to learn, it is equally crucial to consider the diverse patient populations that radiographers encounter. We navigate students through the considerations they need to keep in mind when imaging patients with special needs, such as pediatric, geriatric, and pregnant patients. Each patient population comes with its unique challenges and requirements, and our study materials provide students with the knowledge and skills to address these needs sensitively and effectively.

In addition to the technical instructions, our study guide goes beyond the basics, instilling in students a deep understanding of the rationale behind each procedure. We explain the clinical indications for thorax and abdomen imaging, elaborating on the pathologies, injuries, and conditions that necessitate these procedures. By developing this comprehensive knowledge, students will not only excel in their exams but also be better prepared to make informed decisions in real-life clinical scenarios.

At Test Treasure Publication, we believe that true success lies in fostering a community of learners. Our study materials act as both mentors and companions, inviting students to actively engage with the content, ask questions, and seek enlightenment. We encourage students to interact with fellow learners, forming study groups, and exchanging ideas and experiences.

So whether you are a novice radiography student or a seasoned professional seeking to enhance your skills, our study guide on thorax and abdomen procedures will accompany you on this enlightening journey. Together, let us unravel the wonders of this field, one step at a time, as we illuminate the path to extraordinary success.

Extremity Procedures

To start with, let us delve into the positioning techniques for extremity procedures. For the upper limbs, positioning plays a crucial role in capturing high-quality images. Our study guide will walk you through the proper alignment of the hand, wrist, forearm, elbow, and shoulder, ensuring that each anatomical structure is clearly visualized. With step-by-step instructions and visual aids, we will guide you in achieving optimal positioning for various projections such as the PA, lateral, oblique, and special views.

Similarly, when it comes to lower limb procedures, our guide will provide you with the expertise needed to capture detailed images of the foot, ankle, leg, knee, and hip. From positioning the patient correctly to adjusting the exposure factors, our study materials will equip you with the knowledge and skills required to excel in this field. We will cover projections like the AP, lateral, oblique, and specialized views, ensuring that you have a comprehensive understanding of each procedure.

Exposure factors are another crucial aspect of extremity procedures, and our study guide will leave no stone unturned. We will provide you with the necessary knowledge to determine the appropriate techniques for obtaining optimal radiographic images. Understanding factors such as kilovolts peak (kVp), milliamperes (mA), and exposure time will allow you to adjust the settings based on patient-specific considerations and desired image quality.

Additionally, our guide will delve into the special considerations for pediatric and geriatric patients undergoing extremity procedures. As we know, imaging these populations requires a different approach due to their unique anatomical characteristics and potential health conditions. With our expertise and attention to detail, we will empower you to adapt the positioning techniques and exposure factors according to the specific needs of these patients, ensuring accurate and safe imaging.

At Test Treasure Publication, we believe that success lies in going beyond the ordinary. Our comprehensive study materials will not only equip you with the technical knowledge required for extremity procedures but also provide you with the insight and understanding needed to excel in your future radiography career. Allow us to illuminate the path to extraordinary success, and join us on this journey of profound learning. Together, we will transcend ordinary radiography education and embrace the boundless opportunities that lie ahead.

5.1 Full-Length Practice Test 1

Section 1: Patient Care

1. Ethical and Legal Aspects

Question 1: What is the term for obtaining permission from the patient before conducting a radiologic exam?

A) Legal consent

B) Implied contract

C) Informed consent

D) Verbal agreement

2. Interpersonal Communication

Question 2: Which type of question is best for gathering detailed information from patients?

A) Closed-ended

B) Leading

C) Open-ended

D) Multiple-choice

3. Physical Assistance and Monitoring

Question 3: What device is primarily used to monitor a patient's heart rate and rhythm?

A) Spirometer

B) Electrocardiogram (ECG)

C) Pulse oximeter

D) Sphygmomanometer

4. Medical Emergencies

Question 4: In case of an allergic reaction to contrast media, which medication is commonly administered?

A) Aspirin

B) Epinephrine

C) Ibuprofen

D) Acetaminophen

5. Infection Control

Question 5: What is the best method for preventing the spread of infectious diseases in radiology departments?

A) Antibiotics

B) Hand hygiene

C) Air purifiers

D) UV lights

6. Handling and Disposal of Toxic or Hazardous Material

Question 6: Which organization sets the guidelines for handling radiographic contrast media?

A) FDA
B) EPA
C) OSHA
D) CDC

7. Pharmacology

Question 7: Which of the following medications is a muscle relaxant commonly used during radiologic procedures?

A) Diazepam
B) Paracetamol
C) Furosemide
D) Amoxicillin

Section 2: Safety

8. Principles of Radiation Physics

Question 8: Which of the following best describes the process by which X-rays are produced?

A) Photon absorption
B) Thermal agitation
C) Bremsstrahlung radiation
D) Elastic scattering

9. Biological Aspects of Radiation

Question 9: What is the unit used to measure the biological effect of ionizing radiation?

A) Gray
B) Sievert
C) Roentgen
D) Curie

10. Minimizing Patient Exposure

Question 10: Which technique is effective for minimizing patient exposure during a radiographic exam?

A) Increasing the exposure time
B) Decreasing the distance from the source
C) Collimation
D) Increasing the tube current

11. Personnel Protection (ALARA)

Question 11: What does the acronym ALARA stand for?

A) As Low As Relatively Achievable
B) As Low As Reasonably Achievable
C) As Limited As Reasonably Achievable
D) As Low As Radiologically Achievable

Section 3: Image Production

12. Image Acquisition and Technical Evaluation

Question 12: Which of the following factors primarily affects the spatial resolution of an X-ray image?

A) Exposure time

B) Focal-spot size

C) Tube current

D) Distance from the source

13. Equipment Operation and Quality Assurance

Question 13: What is the primary function of the anode in an X-ray tube?

A) Produce electrons

B) Convert electrons into X-rays

C) Limit the X-ray beam

D) Insulate the tube

Section 4: Procedures

14. Head, Spine, and Pelvis Procedures

Question 14: For a lateral skull X-ray, what is the optimal angle for patient head tilt?

A) 15 degrees

B) 30 degrees

C) 45 degrees

D) 60 degrees

15. Thorax and Abdomen Procedures

Question 15: What is the most commonly used position for a chest X-ray?

A) Supine

B) Prone

C) Upright

D) Lateral

16. Extremity Procedures

Question 16: Which type of fracture is best visualized using an oblique projection?

A) Comminuted

B) Spiral

C) Transverse

D) Avulsion

Section 1: Patient Care

17. Ethical and Legal Aspects

Question 17: Which of the following is an example of a violation of patient confidentiality?

A) Discussing a patient's condition with authorized healthcare providers

B) Refusing to share patient information without consent

C) Talking about a patient's diagnosis in the elevator

D) Seeking informed consent before an invasive procedure

18. Interpersonal Communication

Question 18: What communication barrier can occur when a patient is hearing impaired?

A) Emotional barrier

B) Physical barrier

C) Semantic barrier

D) Cultural barrier

19. Physical Assistance and Monitoring

Question 19: Which of the following devices is commonly used to measure blood pressure?

A) Spirometer

B) Electrocardiogram (ECG)

C) Pulse oximeter

D) Sphygmomanometer

20. Medical Emergencies

Question 20: What should be your first response if a patient faints during a procedure?

A) Leave the room to get help

B) Continue the procedure

C) Elevate the patient's legs

D) Administer medication

21. Infection Control

Question 21: Which type of isolation is used for patients with airborne diseases?

A) Droplet precautions

B) Contact precautions

C) Airborne isolation

D) Standard precautions

22. Handling and Disposal of Toxic or Hazardous Material

Question 22: How should a spill of contrast media be cleaned up?

A) Wipe with a dry cloth

B) Flush with water

C) Use a spill kit

D) Use hand sanitizer

23. Pharmacology

Question 23: Which of the following drugs is commonly used as an anticoagulant during radiologic procedures?

A) Diazepam

B) Heparin

C) Ibuprofen

D) Atropine

Section 2: Safety

24. Principles of Radiation Physics

Question 24: What is the main function of the collimator in X-ray imaging?

A) To filter the X-ray beam

B) To focus the X-ray beam

C) To amplify the X-ray beam

D) To diverge the X-ray beam

25. Biological Aspects of Radiation

Question 25: Which cells are most sensitive to radiation?

A) Nerve cells

B) Muscle cells

C) Red blood cells

D) Epithelial cells

26. Minimizing Patient Exposure

Question 26: Which of the following techniques can help reduce motion blur in pediatric imaging?

A) Use a faster film speed

B) Increase the exposure time

C) Use immobilization devices

D) Increase the kVp

27. Personnel Protection (ALARA)

Question 27: Which of the following is NOT a cardinal principle of radiation protection?

A) Time

B) Distance

C) Shielding

D) Amplification

Section 3: Image Production

28. Image Acquisition and Technical Evaluation

Question 28: What type of artifact appears as a white streak in a CT scan?

A) Beam hardening

B) Aliasing

C) Motion artifact

D) Ring artifact

29. Equipment Operation and Quality Assurance

Question 29: Which quality assurance test checks the uniformity of the CT scanner?

A) Linearity test

B) Resolution test

C) Uniformity test

D) Sensitometry test

Section 4: Procedures

30. Head, Spine, and Pelvis Procedures

Question 30: What is the optimal SID (Source-to-Image Distance) for a lumbar spine X-ray?

A) 40 inches

B) 72 inches

C) 100 inches

D) 60 inches

31. Thorax and Abdomen Procedures

Question 31: Which position is best for visualizing the diaphragm in a chest X-ray?

A) AP erect

B) Lateral decubitus

C) PA

D) AP supine

32. Extremity Procedures

Question 32: Which X-ray view is best for visualizing a Colles' fracture?

A) AP wrist

B) Lateral wrist

C) Oblique wrist

D) PA wrist

Section 1: Patient Care

33. Ethical and Legal Aspects
Question 33: What does the acronym HIPAA stand for?

A) Health Insurance Probable Act

B) Hospital In-Patient Admission Act

C) Health Insurance Portability and Accountability Act

D) Hospital Insurance and Protection Act

34. Interpersonal Communication
Question 34: Which of the following communication skills is essential for explaining procedures to patients?

A) Paraphrasing

B) Active listening

C) Clarification

D) Summarization

35. Physical Assistance and Monitoring
Question 35: What is the normal range for adult respiration?

A) 12-18 breaths per minute

B) 18-22 breaths per minute

C) 8-12 breaths per minute

D) 22-28 breaths per minute

36. Medical Emergencies

Question 36: What should be used to treat an allergic reaction to iodinated contrast media?

A) Antibiotics

B) Antihistamines

C) Antacids

D) Aspirin

37. Infection Control

Question 37: Which of the following is the most effective method for hand hygiene?

A) Soap and water

B) Hand sanitizer

C) Disposable gloves

D) Wet wipes

38. Handling and Disposal of Toxic or Hazardous Material

Question 38: Which federal agency regulates the disposal of medical waste?

A) FDA

B) CDC

C) EPA

D) OSHA

39. Pharmacology

Question 39: Which type of medication is used for pain relief during radiologic procedures?

A) Antipyretics

B) Analgesics

C) Antispasmodics

D) Antihypertensives

Section 2: Safety

40. Principles of Radiation Physics

Question 40: What is the unit of radiation dose in radiography?

A) Curie

B) Becquerel

C) Gray

D) Roentgen

41. Biological Aspects of Radiation

Question 41: Which tissue is least sensitive to radiation?

A) Bone

B) Muscle

C) Brain

D) Intestine

42. Minimizing Patient Exposure

Question 42: What is the purpose of a lead apron in radiography?

A) To protect the patient from electrical hazards

B) To keep the patient warm

C) To reduce scatter radiation

D) To improve image quality

43. Personnel Protection (ALARA)

Question 43: What does ALARA stand for?

A) Always Leave All Radiation Aside

B) As Low As Reasonably Achievable

C) All Local Areas Require Attention

D) Annual Limit on Airborne Radioactivity

Section 3: Image Production

44. Image Acquisition and Technical Evaluation

Question 44: What term is used to describe unwanted exposure on an X-ray image?

A) Overexposure

B) Artifact

C) Noise

D) Ghosting

45. Equipment Operation and Quality Assurance

Question 45: Which of the following tests is conducted to ensure the linearity of an X-ray unit?

A) Spinning top test

B) Sensitometric test

C) Half-value layer test

D) Coin test

Section 4: Procedures

46. Head, Spine, and Pelvis Procedures

Question 46: What position is used for a lateral skull X-ray?

A) Fowler's

B) Sims'

C) Trendelenburg

D) Frankfurt horizontal

47. Thorax and Abdomen Procedures

Question 47: What is the proper technique for an AP abdominal X-ray?

A) Full inspiration

B) Full expiration

C) Partial inspiration

D) Partial expiration

48. Extremity Procedures

Question 48: Which of the following is essential for a knee X-ray?

A) 90-degree flexion of the knee

B) 45-degree flexion of the knee

C) 60-degree flexion of the knee

D) 30-degree flexion of the knee

Section 1: Patient Care

49. Ethical and Legal Aspects

Question 49: Which of the following is an example of an intentional tort in radiography?

A) Battery

B) Negligence

C) Accident

D) Ignorance

50. Interpersonal Communication

Question 50: What is the role of non-verbal communication in patient interaction?

A) Irrelevant

B) Supplementary

C) Detrimental

D) Integral

51. Physical Assistance and Monitoring

Question 51: Which is the most appropriate method for lifting a patient?

A) By their arms

B) Using a mechanical lift

C) With the help of a stretcher

D) Using your back muscles

52. Medical Emergencies

Question 52: How should a radiographer respond to a patient who is choking?

A) Start CPR

B) Use the Heimlich maneuver

C) Administer oxygen

D) Call for a nurse

53. Infection Control

Question 53: What is the minimum percentage of alcohol needed in hand sanitizers to be effective?

A) 40%

B) 50%

C) 60%

D) 70%

54. Handling and Disposal of Toxic or Hazardous Material

Question 54: Which color-coded container is used for sharps disposal?

A) Yellow

B) Red

C) Blue

D) Green

55. Pharmacology

Question 55: Which route of drug administration has the quickest onset of action?

A) Oral

B) Subcutaneous

C) Intramuscular

D) Intravenous

Section 2: Safety

56. Principles of Radiation Physics

Question 56: What does "kVp" stand for in radiography?

A) Kilo-Voltage Peak

B) Kilo-Voltage Pulse

C) Kilo-Velocity Peak

D) Kilo-Variable Pulse

57. Biological Aspects of Radiation

Question 57: Which of the following is most susceptible to radiation damage?

A) Adult cells

B) Somatic cells

C) Germ cells

D) Nerve cells

58. Minimizing Patient Exposure

Question 58: What type of shielding is used to protect the gonads?

A) Lead gloves

B) Collar

C) Flat contact shield

D) Wrap-around apron

59. Personnel Protection (ALARA)

Question 59: What is the maximum permissible dose (MPD) for occupational exposure to radiation?

A) 50 mSv/year

B) 20 mSv/year

C) 100 mSv/year

D) 5 mSv/year

Section 3: Image Production

60. Image Acquisition and Technical Evaluation

Question 60: What type of contrast is ideal for a chest X-ray?

A) High contrast

B) Low contrast

C) Medium contrast

D) No contrast

61. Equipment Operation and Quality Assurance

Question 61: Which type of imaging receptor is sensitive to light?

A) Direct capture

B) Computed radiography

C) Indirect capture

D) Digital radiography

Section 4: Procedures

62. Head, Spine, and Pelvis Procedures

Question 62: Which view is recommended for coccyx imaging?

A) Lateral

B) AP

C) Oblique

D) PA

63. Thorax and Abdomen Procedures

Question 63: Which technique is preferred for imaging the lungs?

A) PA upright

B) AP supine

C) Lateral decubitus

D) Oblique

64. Extremity Procedures

Question 64: What angle should the central ray be for an AP foot X-ray?

A) 5 degrees cephalic

B) 10 degrees cephalic

C) 15 degrees cephalic

D) 20 degrees cephalic

Section 1: Patient Care

65. Ethical and Legal Aspects

Question 65: What is implied consent?

A) Written permission

B) Verbal permission

C) Assumed permission under specific conditions

D) None of the above

66. Interpersonal Communication

Question 66: What is the key component in active listening?

A) Responding

B) Interrupting

C) Multi-tasking

D) Ignoring

67. Physical Assistance and Monitoring

Question 67: What is the most effective way to reduce patient motion during imaging?

A) Use of sedatives

B) Quick exposure

C) Immobilization devices

D) Loud instructions

68. Medical Emergencies

Question 68: What is the first step in the treatment of a burn?

A) Apply ice

B) Rinse with cold water

C) Use antibiotic ointment

D) Apply a bandage

69. Infection Control

Question 69: Which of the following is a contact precaution?

A) Wearing a mask

B) Wearing gloves

C) Eye protection

D) Respirator

70. Handling and Disposal of Toxic or Hazardous Material

Question 70: Which agency sets the guidelines for hazardous waste disposal?

A) FDA

B) EPA

C) CDC

D) WHO

71. Pharmacology

Question 71: Which of the following drugs is a common anticoagulant?

A) Aspirin

B) Warfarin

C) Acetaminophen

D) Amoxicillin

Section 2: Safety

72. Principles of Radiation Physics

Question 72: What is the unit of absorbed radiation dose?

A) Röntgen

B) Curie

C) Gray

D) Becquerel

73. Biological Aspects of Radiation

Question 73: What is the principle behind the ALARA concept?

A) Maximize exposure

B) Minimize exposure

C) Constant exposure

D) Variable exposure

74. Minimizing Patient Exposure

Question 74: What should be the minimum distance from the radiation source during a mobile X-ray?

A) 1 meter

B) 2 meters

C) 3 meters

D) 6 feet

75. Personnel Protection (ALARA)

Question 75: Which of the following materials is most commonly used in radiation shielding?

A) Rubber

B) Plastic

C) Lead

D) Aluminum

Section 3: Image Production

76. Image Acquisition and Technical Evaluation

Question 76: What is the role of a grid in radiography?

A) Reduce exposure

B) Increase contrast

C) Increase resolution

D) Reduce scatter

77. Equipment Operation and Quality Assurance

Question 77: What is the primary purpose of collimation?

A) Increase field size

B) Reduce patient dose

C) Increase image contrast

D) Decrease image resolution

Section 4: Procedures

78. Head, Spine, and Pelvis Procedures

Question 78: Which projection is commonly used for cervical spine imaging?

A) AP

B) Lateral

C) Oblique

D) PA

79. Thorax and Abdomen Procedures

Question 79: What is the optimal position for a lateral chest X-ray?

A) Arms crossed

B) Hands on hips

C) Arms raised

D) Hands clasped behind the head

80. Extremity Procedures

Question 80: What is the main advantage of using MRI over X-ray for soft tissue imaging?

A) Lower cost

B) Higher resolution

C) Lower radiation exposure

D) Faster imaging time

Section 1: Patient Care

81. Ethical and Legal Aspects

Question 81: Which of the following documents protects patient confidentiality?

A) Good Samaritan Law

B) HIPAA

C) Medical Power of Attorney

D) Informed Consent Form

82. Interpersonal Communication

Question 82: What is nonverbal communication?

A) Writing

B) Speech

C) Body language

D) Email

83. Physical Assistance and Monitoring

Question 83: Which vital sign is typically measured by a sphygmomanometer?

A) Blood Pressure

B) Heart Rate

C) Respiratory Rate

D) Temperature

84. Medical Emergencies

Question 84: What is the immediate treatment for anaphylaxis?

A) Insulin

B) Antacid

C) Epinephrine

D) Aspirin

85. Infection Control

Question 85: What is the recommended handwashing duration according to the CDC?

A) 10 seconds

B) 20 seconds

C) 30 seconds

D) 60 seconds

86. Handling and Disposal of Toxic or Hazardous Material

Question 86: How should broken glass be disposed of in a healthcare setting?

A) Regular trash

B) Sharps container

C) Recycle bin

D) Biohazard waste bag

87. Pharmacology

Question 87: Which drug is commonly used for pain relief?

A) Insulin

B) Ibuprofen

C) Penicillin

D) Warfarin

Section 2: Safety

88. Principles of Radiation Physics

Question 88: What is the primary function of an X-ray tube anode?

A) Generate electrons

B) Convert electrons to X-rays

C) Block X-rays

D) Collimate X-rays

89. Biological Aspects of Radiation

Question 89: What is the stochastic effect of radiation?

A) Immediate skin burn

B) Tissue necrosis

C) Cancer risk

D) Cataract formation

90. Minimizing Patient Exposure

Question 90: Which technique can help reduce motion artifacts in pediatric radiography?

A) Increase exposure time

B) Parental involvement

C) Reduce kVp

D) Use a grid

91. Personnel Protection (ALARA)

Question 91: What should be done immediately after a radiation exposure incident?

A) Evacuate the area

B) Notify the Radiation Safety Officer

C) Decontaminate the area

D) Wait for symptoms

Section 3: Image Production

92. Image Acquisition and Technical Evaluation

Question 92: What does a high signal-to-noise ratio (SNR) indicate?

A) Poor image quality

B) Good image quality

C) Overexposure

D) Underexposure

93. Equipment Operation and Quality Assurance

Question 93: Which quality control test should be performed daily?

A) Beam alignment

B) Collimator accuracy

C) Focal spot size

D) Automatic exposure control (AEC)

Section 4: Procedures

94. Head, Spine, and Pelvis Procedures
Question 94: Which view is most suitable for imaging the occipital bone?

A) AP

B) PA

C) Towne view

D) Lateral

95. Thorax and Abdomen Procedures
Question 95: What is the breathing instruction for a standard PA chest X-ray?

A) Inhale and hold

B) Exhale and hold

C) Normal breathing

D) None

96. Extremity Procedures
Question 96: Which modality is ideal for imaging complex fractures?

A) CT

B) MRI

C) Ultrasound

D) Standard X-ray

Additional Questions

97. Advanced Imaging Modalities

Question 97: Which imaging modality is best suited for visualizing soft tissue contrast?

A) MRI

B) CT

C) X-Ray

D) Ultrasound

98. General Anatomy and Positioning Principles

Question 98: What does the term "oblique" imply in radiographic positioning?

A) Lateral rotation

B) No rotation

C) Posterior to Anterior

D) Anterior to Posterior

99. Data Management

Question 99: Which file format is commonly used for medical images in radiography?

A) JPEG

B) DICOM

C) PNG

D) BMP

100. Patient Preparation and Safety

Question 100: What should be removed before performing an MRI scan?

A) Clothing

B) Metallic objects

C) Glasses

D) All of the above

5.2 Answer Sheet - Practice Test 1

1. Answer: C) Informed consent

Explanation: Informed consent refers to the process of providing all relevant information about the procedure to the patient and obtaining their permission to proceed.

2. Answer: C) Open-ended

Explanation: Open-ended questions encourage a more comprehensive response, providing an opportunity to gather detailed information from the patient.

3. Answer: B) Electrocardiogram (ECG)

Explanation: An ECG is used to monitor the electrical activity of the heart, providing information on heart rate and rhythm.

4. Answer: B) Epinephrine

Explanation: Epinephrine is often used to treat severe allergic reactions and anaphylaxis, commonly caused by contrast media.

5. Answer: B) Hand hygiene

Explanation: Hand hygiene is the most effective method to prevent the transmission of infections in healthcare settings.

6. Answer: A) FDA

Explanation: The Food and Drug Administration (FDA) sets the guidelines for the safe handling and disposal of radiographic contrast media.

7. Answer: A) Diazepam

Explanation: Diazepam is a muscle relaxant often used to reduce patient discomfort during certain radiologic procedures.

8. Answer: C) Bremsstrahlung radiation

Explanation: Bremsstrahlung radiation is the primary process through which X-rays are generated in an X-ray tube.

9. Answer: B) Sievert

Explanation: Sievert is the unit that measures the biological effect of ionizing radiation on human tissue.

10. Answer: C) Collimation

Explanation: Collimation helps to focus the X-ray beam on the specific area of interest, thereby minimizing exposure to surrounding tissues.

11. Answer: B) As Low As Reasonably Achievable

Explanation: ALARA stands for "As Low As Reasonably Achievable," a principle designed to minimize radiation exposure to patients and healthcare providers.

12. Answer: B) Focal-spot size

Explanation: The size of the focal spot is a significant factor in determining the spatial resolution of an X-ray image.

13. Answer: B) Convert electrons into X-rays

Explanation: The anode serves as the target for electrons, converting them into X-ray photons.

14. Answer: A) 15 degrees

Explanation: A 15-degree head tilt is generally recommended for optimal imaging of the lateral skull.

15. Answer: C) Upright

Explanation: The upright position is most commonly used for chest X-rays, as it allows for optimal lung expansion and clear imaging.

16. Answer: B) Spiral

Explanation: A spiral fracture is best visualized using an oblique projection, which offers a more detailed view of the fracture pattern.

17. Answer: C) Talking about a patient's diagnosis in the elevator

Explanation: Discussing a patient's diagnosis in public spaces like an elevator violates patient confidentiality and should be avoided.

18. Answer: B) Physical barrier

Explanation: A physical barrier to communication occurs when there are physiological limitations, such as hearing impairment.

19. Answer: D) Sphygmomanometer

Explanation: A sphygmomanometer is commonly used to measure blood pressure by evaluating the pressure exerted on the walls of the arteries.

20. Answer: C) Elevate the patient's legs

Explanation: If a patient faints, elevating their legs can help restore proper blood flow to the brain.

21. Answer: C) Airborne isolation

Explanation: Airborne isolation is used for patients with diseases that are transmitted through the air, such as tuberculosis.

22. Answer: C) Use a spill kit

Explanation: A spill kit containing absorbent material and protective equipment should be used to clean up spills of contrast media safely.

23. Answer: B) Heparin

Explanation: Heparin is an anticoagulant that prevents blood clotting and is often used during radiologic procedures that require vascular access.

24. Answer: B) To focus the X-ray beam

Explanation: The collimator focuses the X-ray beam on the area of interest, reducing scatter radiation and improving image quality.

25. Answer: D) Epithelial cells

Explanation: Epithelial cells, which line organs and form skin, are generally more sensitive to radiation due to their rapid rate of division.

26. Answer: C) Use immobilization devices

Explanation: Using immobilization devices can help keep pediatric patients still during the exposure, reducing motion blur.

27. Answer: D) Amplification

Explanation: The cardinal principles of radiation protection are time, distance, and shielding. Amplification is not one of them.

28. Answer: A) Beam hardening

Explanation: Beam hardening artifacts appear as white streaks in CT images and are caused by the differential absorption of low- and high-energy photons.

29. Answer: C) Uniformity test

Explanation: The uniformity test checks for consistent image quality across the field of view in a CT scanner.

30. Answer: B) 72 inches

Explanation: A SID of 72 inches is optimal for a lumbar spine X-ray to reduce magnification and improve image quality.

31. Answer: A) AP erect

Explanation: The AP erect position allows for optimal visualization of the diaphragm and lungs in a chest X-ray.

32. Answer: A) AP wrist

Explanation: The AP wrist view is generally considered the best for visualizing a Colles' fracture, which occurs at the distal radius near the wrist.

33. Answer: C) Health Insurance Portability and Accountability Act

Explanation: HIPAA stands for Health Insurance Portability and Accountability Act, which regulates the privacy and security of patient information.

34. Answer: C) Clarification

Explanation: Clarification is essential when explaining procedures to patients to ensure that they fully understand what to expect.

35. Answer: A) 12-18 breaths per minute

Explanation: The normal range for adult respiration is 12-18 breaths per minute.

36. Answer: B) Antihistamines

Explanation: Antihistamines are commonly used to treat allergic reactions to iodinated contrast media.

37. Answer: A) Soap and water

Explanation: Soap and water are considered the most effective methods for hand hygiene, particularly for removing certain types of microbes.

38. Answer: C) EPA

Explanation: The Environmental Protection Agency (EPA) regulates the disposal of medical waste.

39. Answer: B) Analgesics

Explanation: Analgesics are used for pain relief during radiologic procedures.

40. Answer: C) Gray

Explanation: The unit of radiation dose in radiography is Gray (Gy).

41. Answer: A) Bone

Explanation: Bone tissue is least sensitive to radiation due to its lower metabolic rate compared to other tissues.

42. Answer: C) To reduce scatter radiation

Explanation: The lead apron is used to reduce scatter radiation and protect areas of the patient's body that are not being imaged.

43. Answer: B) As Low As Reasonably Achievable

Explanation: ALARA stands for "As Low As Reasonably Achievable," a principle aimed at minimizing radiation exposure.

44. Answer: B) Artifact

Explanation: Artifacts are unwanted exposures that can interfere with the interpretation of an X-ray image.

45. Answer: A) Spinning top test

Explanation: The spinning top test is used to ensure that the X-ray unit is operating in a linear fashion.

46. Answer: D) Frankfurt horizontal

Explanation: The Frankfurt horizontal position is commonly used for lateral skull X-rays to ensure proper alignment and image quality.

47. Answer: B) Full expiration

Explanation: A full expiration is recommended for an AP abdominal X-ray to properly visualize abdominal structures.

48. Answer: B) 45-degree flexion of the knee

Explanation: A 45-degree flexion of the knee is essential for most standard knee X-rays to get optimal imaging.

49. Answer: A) Battery

Explanation: Battery is an example of an intentional tort in radiography. It involves touching a patient without their informed consent.

50. Answer: D) Integral

Explanation: Non-verbal communication is integral to patient interaction as it can convey important emotional and contextual information.

51. Answer: B) Using a mechanical lift

Explanation: Using a mechanical lift is the most appropriate and safest method for lifting a patient to minimize the risk of injury.

52. Answer: B) Use the Heimlich maneuver

Explanation: If a patient is choking, the Heimlich maneuver is the appropriate immediate response to dislodge the obstructing item.

53. Answer: C) 60%

Explanation: The minimum percentage of alcohol needed for hand sanitizers to be effective is 60%.

54. Answer: B) Red

Explanation: Red color-coded containers are typically used for the disposal of sharps in medical settings.

55. Answer: D) Intravenous

Explanation: Intravenous (IV) administration has the quickest onset of action as it delivers the drug directly into the bloodstream.

56. Answer: A) Kilo-Voltage Peak

Explanation: "KVP" stands for Kilo-Voltage Peak, a unit that sets the quality or penetrating ability of the X-ray beam.

57. Answer: C) Germ cells

Explanation: Germ cells are most susceptible to radiation damage because they are involved in reproduction and have a high rate of division.

58. Answer: C) Flat contact shield

Explanation: A flat contact shield is specifically designed to protect the gonads during radiographic procedures.

59. Answer: A) 50 mSv/year

Explanation: The maximum permissible dose for occupational exposure to radiation is 50 mSv/year according to most guidelines.

60. Answer: A) High contrast

Explanation: High contrast is ideal for a chest X-ray because it allows for better visualization of the structures within the thoracic cavity.

61. Answer: B) Computed radiography

Explanation: Computed radiography uses an imaging plate that is sensitive to light.

62. Answer: A) Lateral

Explanation: A lateral view is recommended for coccyx imaging to get optimal visualization.

63. Answer: A) PA upright

Explanation: PA upright is the preferred technique for lung imaging as it minimizes magnification of the heart.

64. Answer: C) 15 degrees cephalic

Explanation: A 15-degree cephalic angle of the central ray is recommended for an AP foot X-ray for proper image acquisition.

65. Answer: C) Assumed permission under specific conditions

Explanation: Implied consent is assumed under specific conditions, such as when immediate action is required to save a patient's life and the patient is unable to give explicit consent.

66. Answer: A) Responding

Explanation: Responding appropriately is a key component of active listening, as it shows the speaker that you are engaged in the conversation.

67. Answer: C) Immobilization devices

Explanation: Immobilization devices are the most effective way to reduce patient motion during imaging procedures.

68. Answer: B) Rinse with cold water

Explanation: Rinsing the affected area with cold water is the first step in treating a burn, as it helps to cool down the area and minimize tissue damage.

69. Answer: B) Wearing gloves

Explanation: Wearing gloves is a contact precaution aimed at preventing the direct transfer of pathogens.

70. Answer: B) EPA

Explanation: The Environmental Protection Agency (EPA) sets the guidelines for the handling and disposal of hazardous waste.

71. Answer: B) Warfarin

Explanation: Warfarin is a common anticoagulant used to prevent blood clots.

72. Answer: C) Gray

Explanation: The unit of absorbed radiation dose is Gray (Gy).

73. Answer: B) Minimize exposure

Explanation: The principle behind ALARA (As Low As Reasonably Achievable) is to minimize radiation exposure to both patients and healthcare workers.

74. Answer: D) 6 feet

Explanation: The minimum safe distance from the radiation source during a mobile X-ray should be at least 6 feet to minimize exposure.

75. Answer: C) Lead

Explanation: Lead is most commonly used in radiation shielding because of its high atomic number, which effectively attenuates X-rays.

76. Answer: D) Reduce scatter

Explanation: The grid is used in radiography to reduce scatter radiation, thereby improving image quality.

77. Answer: B) Reduce patient dose

Explanation: The primary purpose of collimation is to reduce the patient's radiation dose by limiting the field size.

78. Answer: B) Lateral

Explanation: A lateral projection is commonly used for cervical spine imaging as it provides better visualization of the vertebrae.

79. Answer: C) Arms raised

Explanation: Arms should be raised for a lateral chest X-ray to remove the arms and shoulders from the field of view.

80. Answer: B) Higher resolution

Explanation: MRI offers higher resolution for soft tissue imaging compared to X-ray, making it ideal for detailed analysis.

81. Answer: B) HIPAA

Explanation: HIPAA (Health Insurance Portability and Accountability Act) protects patient confidentiality by setting standards for the protection of medical information.

82. Answer: C) Body language

Explanation: Nonverbal communication involves the use of body language, gestures, and facial expressions to convey information or emotions.

83. Answer: A) Blood Pressure

Explanation: A sphygmomanometer is used to measure blood pressure, an essential vital sign in monitoring a patient's health.

84. Answer: C) Epinephrine

Explanation: Epinephrine is the immediate treatment for anaphylaxis and is typically administered via an auto-injector.

85. Answer: B) 20 seconds

Explanation: The CDC recommends washing hands for at least 20 seconds to effectively remove germs.

86. Answer: B) Sharps container

Explanation: Broken glass should be disposed of in a sharps container to prevent injury.

87. Answer: B) Ibuprofen

Explanation: Ibuprofen is a common over-the-counter drug used for pain relief.

88. Answer: B) Convert electrons to X-rays

Explanation: The primary function of an X-ray tube anode is to convert high-speed electrons into X-rays.

89. Answer: C) Cancer risk

Explanation: Stochastic effects, such as an increased risk of cancer, are long-term effects that may occur after exposure to radiation.

90. Answer: B) Parental involvement

Explanation: Parental involvement can help calm the child and reduce motion, thereby reducing the likelihood of artifacts.

91. Answer: B) Notify the Radiation Safety Officer

Explanation: Any radiation exposure incident should be immediately reported to the Radiation Safety Officer for appropriate action.

92. Answer: B) Good image quality

Explanation: A high SNR indicates good image quality by showing that the signal is much greater than the background noise.

93. Answer: B) Collimator accuracy

Explanation: Daily checks of collimator accuracy ensure that the radiation field is well-defined and aligned.

94. Answer: C) Towne view

Explanation: The Towne view is specifically designed for better visualization of the occipital bone.

95. Answer: A) Inhale and hold

Explanation: For a standard PA chest X-ray, the patient is usually instructed to inhale and hold their breath to ensure optimal imaging conditions.

96. Answer: A) CT

Explanation: CT scans are ideal for imaging complex fractures as they offer detailed cross-sectional images.

97. Answer: A) MRI

Explanation: MRI (Magnetic Resonance Imaging) is best suited for visualizing soft tissue contrast as it provides excellent spatial resolution and can differentiate between various soft tissues.

98. Answer: A) Lateral rotation

Explanation: The term "oblique" in radiographic positioning indicates that there is some lateral rotation involved, showing the structure of interest from an angle.

99. Answer: B) DICOM

Explanation: DICOM (Digital Imaging and Communications in Medicine) is a standardized file format and network protocol used for storing and transmitting medical images.

100. Answer: D) All of the above

Explanation: Before undergoing an MRI scan, all metallic objects, glasses, and clothing (often replaced by a hospital gown) should be removed to ensure patient safety and optimal image quality.

6.1 FULL-LENGTH PRACTICE TEST 2

Section 1: The Patient Care

101. Ethical and Legal Aspects

Question 101: Which of the following principles requires radiologic technologists to "do no harm"?

A) Beneficence

B) Nonmaleficence

C) Autonomy

D) Justice

102. Interpersonal Communication

Question 102:

What is the best approach when explaining a radiologic procedure to a child?

A) Use technical jargon

B) Use simple language and props

C) Explain only to the parent

D) Avoid explanation to minimize anxiety

103. Physical Assistance and Monitoring

Question 103:

Which device monitors a patient's heart rate and rhythm?

A) Blood Pressure Cuff

B) Pulse Oximeter

C) ECG

D) Thermometer

104. Medical Emergencies

Question 104:

What is the first aid for a radiology patient who faints?

A) Give water

B) Lay them flat and elevate the legs

C) Apply cold compress

D) Call for a stretcher

105. Infection Control

Question 105:

Which method of sterilization uses steam?

A) Dry heat

B) Autoclaving

C) Chemical sterilization

D) Gas sterilization

106. Handling and Disposal of Toxic or Hazardous Material

Question 106:

How should a radiologic technologist dispose of used sharps?

A) In the general trash bin

B) In a biohazard container

C) In a paper bag

D) In a sharps container

107. Pharmacology

Question 107:

Which type of drug is typically used to relax patients before an MRI?

A) Antacid

B) Sedative

C) Antibiotic

D) Antipyretic

Section 2: The Safety

108. Principles of Radiation Physics

Question 108:

Which particle is ejected in beta decay?

A) Neutron

B) Proton

C) Electron

D) Alpha particle

109. Biological Aspects of Radiation

Question 109:

What does the term "radiosensitive" imply?

A) Resistance to radiation

B) Attraction to radiation

C) Sensitivity to radiation

D) Insensitivity to radiation

110. Minimizing Patient Exposure

Question 110:

Which of the following is not a cardinal rule of radiation protection?

A) Time

B) Distance

C) Shielding

D) Magnification

111. Personnel Protection (ALARA)

Question 111:

What does ALARA stand for?

A) As Low As Reasonably Achievable

B) As Long As Really Available

C) After Last Authorized Radiograph

D) Average Lifetime Adult Radiation Allowance

Section 3: The Image Production

112. Image Acquisition and Technical Evaluation

Question 112:

What affects the contrast of an X-ray image?

A) Tube current

B) Tube voltage

C) Exposure time

D) Anode material

113. Equipment Operation and Quality Assurance

Question 113:

Which test ensures the X-ray beam is aligned with the image receptor?

A) Collimator test

B) Beam alignment test

C) Focal spot size test

D) Tube warm-up

Section 4: The Procedures

114. Head, Spine, and Pelvis Procedures

Question 114:

Which radiographic projection is used to visualize the cervical spine?

A) AP

B) PA

C) Lateral

D) Oblique

115. Thorax and Abdomen Procedures

Question 115:

What is the standard exposure time for a chest X-ray?

A) 1/60 second

B) 1/30 second

C) 1/120 second

D) 1/180 second

116. Extremity Procedures

Question 116:

Which view of the hand would show a Bennett's fracture?

A) PA

B) Oblique

C) Lateral

D) AP

Section 1: The Patient Care

117. Ethical and Legal Aspects

Question 117:

Which of the following is an example of an intentional tort in radiology?

A) Battery

B) Negligence

C) Misdiagnosis

D) Malpractice

118. Interpersonal Communication

Question 118:

Active listening involves:

A) Talking while the patient is speaking

B) Offering advice immediately

C) Ignoring non-verbal cues

D) Paraphrasing and asking clarifying questions

119. Physical Assistance and Monitoring

Question 119:

Which of the following vitals is typically the last to change in a deteriorating patient?

A) Heart rate

B) Blood pressure

C) Respiratory rate

D) Temperature

120. Medical Emergencies

Question 120:

In the event of a fire, what does the acronym RACE stand for?

A) Run, Alert, Call, Extinguish

B) Rescue, Alarm, Contain, Extinguish

C) Run, Activate, Cover, Extinguish

D) Rescue, Alert, Cover, Evacuate

121. Infection Control

Question 121:

What is the minimum percentage of alcohol required for an effective hand sanitizer?

A) 40%

B) 50%

C) 60%

D) 70%

122. Handling and Disposal of Toxic or Hazardous Material

Question 122:

How often should eyewash stations be checked?

A) Daily

B) Weekly

C) Monthly

D) Annually

123. Pharmacology

Question 123:

What is the reversal agent for an opioid overdose?

A) Epinephrine

B) Naloxone

C) Atropine

D) Flumazenil

Section 2: The Safety

124. Principles of Radiation Physics

Question 124:

Which type of interaction with matter involves the ejection of a K-shell electron?

A) Coherent scattering

B) Compton scattering

C) Photoelectric effect

D) Pair production

125. Biological Aspects of Radiation

Question 125:

What is the SI unit for measuring radiation dose?

A) Roentgen

B) Rad

C) Gray

D) Curie

126. Minimizing Patient Exposure

Question 126:

Which of the following techniques can be used to minimize motion blur?

A) Increase exposure time

B) Decrease tube current

C) Use a grid

D) Use a higher speed image receptor

127. Personnel Protection (ALARA)

Question 127:

What is the annual dose limit for radiation workers?

A) 10 mSv

B) 50 mSv

C) 20 mSv

D) 5 mSv

Section 3: The Image Production

128. Image Acquisition and Technical Evaluation

Question 128:

What determines the spatial resolution of an image?

A) kVp

B) mAs

C) Pixel size

D) Exposure time

129. Equipment Operation and Quality Assurance

Question 129:

What is the primary purpose of a collimator?

A) To focus the X-ray beam

B) To filter the X-ray beam

C) To reduce patient exposure

D) To intensify the image

Section 4: The Procedures

130. Head, Spine, and Pelvis Procedures

Question 130:

Which technique is best for imaging the skull sutures?

A) AP

B) PA

C) Lateral

D) Tangential

131. Thorax and Abdomen Procedures

Question 131:

Which modality is most effective for imaging soft tissue in the abdomen?

A) X-ray

B) MRI

C) CT

D) Ultrasound

132. Extremity Procedures

Question 132:

Which X-ray view is recommended for a suspected scaphoid fracture?

A) PA

B) Lateral

C) Oblique

D) Ulnar deviation

Section 1: The Patient Care

133. Ethical and Legal Aspects

Question 133:

Which of the following best defines the term "informed consent"?

A) Oral agreement to treatment

B) Written agreement to treatment without understanding it

C) Written agreement to treatment after understanding risks and benefits

D) Ignoring patient's queries about treatment

134. Interpersonal Communication

Question 134:

Which of the following is a form of non-verbal communication?

A) Texting

B) Nodding

C) Whispering

D) E-mailing

135. Physical Assistance and Monitoring

Question 135:

What does the Glasgow Coma Scale assess?

A) Pain

B) Respiratory rate

C) Neurological status

D) Blood pressure

136. Medical Emergencies

Question 136:

What is the first action when someone is suspected of having a stroke?

A) Give them water

B) Perform CPR

C) Call 911

D) Administer aspirin

137. Infection Control

Question 137:

Which method is best for sterilization of surgical instruments?

A) Boiling water

B) Autoclave

C) Soap and water

D) UV light

138. Handling and Disposal of Toxic or Hazardous Material
Question 138:

What color coding is used for biohazard waste?

A) Green

B) Yellow

C) Red

D) Blue

139. Pharmacology
Question 139:

Which drug is a common vasodilator?

A) Nitroglycerin

B) Atropine

C) Furosemide

D) Epinephrine

Section 2: The Safety

140. Principles of Radiation Physics

Question 140:

What happens to the image quality when the kVp is increased?

A) Increases

B) Decreases

C) Remains the same

D) Becomes blurry

141. Biological Aspects of Radiation

Question 141:

What is the principal effect of ionizing radiation on human tissue?

A) Mechanical damage

B) Thermal injury

C) Genetic mutations

D) Electrical imbalance

142. Minimizing Patient Exposure

Question 142:

How can you minimize radiation scatter?

A) Using lower kVp

B) Increasing distance from the source

C) Removing lead shields

D) Increasing the beam size

143. Personnel Protection (ALARA)

Question 143:

What does ALARA stand for?

A) As Long As Reasonably Achievable

B) As Low As Reasonably Achievable

C) As Low As Really Allowed

D) As Long As Really Achievable

Section 3: The Image Production

144. Image Acquisition and Technical Evaluation

Question 144:

Which of the following artifacts can be caused by patient motion?

A) Vignetting

B) Blurring

C) Dead pixels

D) Ghosting

145. Equipment Operation and Quality Assurance

Question 145:

What type of quality assurance test ensures that the X-ray beam is aligned properly?

A) Light field test

B) Dosimetry

C) Spatial resolution test

D) Focal spot size test

Section 4: The Procedures

146. Head, Spine, and Pelvis Procedures

Question 146:

What is the standard imaging study for a suspected pelvic fracture?

A) AP pelvic X-ray

B) CT scan

C) MRI

D) Ultrasound

147. Thorax and Abdomen Procedures

Question 147:

What is the modality of choice for staging lung cancer?

A) X-ray

B) PET scan

C) CT scan

D) MRI

148. Extremity Procedures

Question 148:

What projection is preferred for imaging the first metatarsophalangeal joint?

A) AP

B) Oblique

C) Lateral

D) Sesamoid

Section 1: The Patient Care

149. Ethical and Legal Aspects

Question 149:

Who is legally authorized to sign a consent form for a minor?

A) Teacher

B) Guardian

C) Neighbor

D) Sibling

150. Interpersonal Communication

Question 150:

What is the purpose of using open-ended questions in patient interviews?

A) Limit responses

B) Encourage brief answers

C) Encourage detailed answers

D) Confuse the patient

151. Physical Assistance and Monitoring

Question 151:

What does the term "tachypnea" refer to?

A) Slow heart rate

B) Rapid breathing

C) High blood pressure

D) Low blood sugar

152. Medical Emergencies

Question 152:

What is the antidote for acetaminophen poisoning?

A) Naloxone

B) Flumazenil

C) N-acetylcysteine

D) Atropine

153. Infection Control

Question 153:

Which type of isolation is used for patients with tuberculosis?

A) Droplet

B) Airborne

C) Contact

D) Standard

154. Handling and Disposal of Toxic or Hazardous Material

Question 154:

What type of fire extinguisher should be used for electrical fires?

A) Class A

B) Class B

C) Class C

D) Class D

155. Pharmacology

Question 155:

Which of the following medications is an anticoagulant?

A) Warfarin

B) Acetaminophen

C) Amoxicillin

D) Hydrocortisone

Section 2: The Safety

156. Principles of Radiation Physics

Question 156:

What does "mAs" stand for in radiography?

A) Milli-Ampere second

B) Mega-Ampere second

C) Micro-Ampere second

D) Mini-Ampere second

157. Biological Aspects of Radiation

Question 157:

Which type of radiation is non-ionizing?

A) X-ray

B) Gamma rays

C) Ultraviolet light

D) Microwave

158. Minimizing Patient Exposure

Question 158:

Which technique can reduce the risk of motion artifacts?

A) Longer exposure time

B) Higher kVp

C) Shorter exposure time

D) Lower mAs

159. Personnel Protection (ALARA)

Question 159:

Which shielding material is commonly used to protect against X-rays?

A) Aluminum

B) Lead

C) Plastic

D) Iron

Section 3: The Image Production

160. Image Acquisition and Technical Evaluation
Question 160:
What is a histogram in digital imaging?

A) Color balance

B) Brightness distribution

C) Sharpness

D) Contrast

161. Equipment Operation and Quality Assurance
Question 161:
What is the purpose of a collimator in radiography?

A) To increase exposure time

B) To restrict the X-ray beam

C) To enhance contrast

D) To increase magnification

Section 4: The Procedures

162. Head, Spine, and Pelvis Procedures
Question 162:
Which imaging modality is contraindicated for patients with pacemakers?

A) CT scan

B) X-ray

C) MRI

D) Ultrasound

163. Thorax and Abdomen Procedures

Question 163:

What is the primary purpose of a barium enema?

A) Detect lung abnormalities

B) Examine the lower gastrointestinal tract

C) Assess kidney function

D) Evaluate the gallbladder

164. Extremity Procedures

Question 164:

Which view is recommended for a lateral wrist radiograph?

A) Pronation

B) Supination

C) Flexion

D) Extension

Section 1: The Patient Care

165. Ethical and Legal Aspects

Question 165:

What is the principle of autonomy in healthcare?

A) Treating everyone equally

B) Making decisions for the patient

C) The right to refuse treatment

D) Act in the patient's best interest

166. Interpersonal Communication

Question 166:

Which non-verbal cue can indicate that a patient is anxious?

A) Smiling

B) Crossed arms

C) Eye contact

D) Nodding

167. Physical Assistance and Monitoring

Question 167:

What device is used to measure blood oxygen saturation?

A) Sphygmomanometer

B) Stethoscope

C) Pulse oximeter

D) ECG machine

168. Medical Emergencies

Question 168:

Which of the following is a symptom of anaphylaxis?

A) Constipation

B) Difficulty breathing

C) Dry mouth

D) Fever

169. Infection Control

Question 169:

Which method is most effective for sterilization?

A) Boiling

B) Autoclaving

C) UV light

D) Alcohol wipes

170. Handling and Disposal of Toxic or Hazardous Material

Question 170:

Where should sharps be disposed of?

A) Regular trash

B) Sharps container

C) Recycle bin

D) Sink disposal

171. Pharmacology

Question 171:

What is the main side effect of diuretics?

A) Constipation

B) Dehydration

C) Drowsiness

D) Nausea

Section 2: The Safety

172. Principles of Radiation Physics

Question 172:

What is the unit of dose equivalent in radiation?

A) Becquerel

B) Sievert

C) Gray

D) Curie

173. Biological Aspects of Radiation

Question 173:

Which cells are most sensitive to radiation?

A) Nerve cells

B) Muscle cells

C) Epithelial cells

D) Blood cells

174. Minimizing Patient Exposure

Question 174:

What does collimation primarily affect in radiography?

A) Contrast

B) Resolution

C) Exposure area

D) Magnification

175. Personnel Protection (ALARA)

Question 175:

What does the acronym ALARA stand for?

A) As Late As Reasonably Achievable

B) As Low As Relatively Achievable

C) As Low As Reasonably Achievable

D) As Long As Reasonably Achievable

Section 3: The Image Production

176. Image Acquisition and Technical Evaluation

Question 176:

Which factor affects image sharpness?

A) kVp

B) mAs

C) Focal spot size

D) Patient thickness

177. Equipment Operation and Quality Assurance

Question 177:

What is the purpose of quality control tests in radiography?

A) To train staff

B) To assess patient satisfaction

C) To validate equipment functionality

D) To reduce costs

Section 4: The Procedures

178. Head, Spine, and Pelvis Procedures

Question 178:

What is the first step in performing a lumbar puncture?

A) Applying local anesthesia

B) Taking a preliminary X-ray

C) Positioning the patient

D) Administering sedation

179. Thorax and Abdomen Procedures

Question 179:

Which view is used to best visualize the diaphragm in chest radiography?

A) AP view

B) PA view

C) Lateral view

D) Oblique view

180. Extremity Procedures

Question 180:

Which bone is commonly fractured in falls involving outstretched hands?

A) Ulna

B) Radius

C) Humerus

D) Scapula

Section 1: The Patient Care

181. Ethical and Legal Aspects

Question 181:

What does the term "informed consent" mean?

A) Verbal agreement to treatment

B) Written agreement to treatment

C) A patient understands the risks, benefits, and alternatives

D) Parental permission for minors

182. Interpersonal Communication

Question 182:

What is the primary purpose of active listening in healthcare?

A) Speeding up consultation

B) Gaining rapport with the patient

C) Ensuring accuracy of information

D) Improving multi-tasking

183. Physical Assistance and Monitoring

Question 183:

Which device is used to monitor heart rate?

A) Spirometer

B) ECG monitor

C) Thermometer

D) Sphygmomanometer

184. Medical Emergencies

Question 184:

What is the first step in the Heimlich maneuver?

A) Giving back blows

B) Calling 911

C) Assessing the patient

D) Standing behind the patient

185. Infection Control

Question 185:

Which method is not effective for sterilization?

A) Boiling

B) Autoclaving

C) Alcohol wipes

D) Dry heat

186. Handling and Disposal of Toxic or Hazardous Material

Question 186:

Which color-coded bin is used for biohazardous waste?

A) Yellow

B) Red

C) Blue

D) Green

187. Pharmacology

Question 187:

Which drug class is commonly used for pain relief?

A) Antibiotics

B) Diuretics

C) Analgesics

D) Antihistamines

Section 2: The Safety

188. Principles of Radiation Physics

Question 188:

Which type of radiation is most harmful to human tissues?

A) Alpha

B) Beta

C) Gamma

D) X-rays

189. Biological Aspects of Radiation

Question 189:

What is the most sensitive phase of the cell cycle to radiation?

A) G1

B) S

C) G2

D) M

190. Minimizing Patient Exposure

Question 190:

What term describes the dose of radiation below which no harmful effects are expected?

A) Dose limit

B) Threshold dose

C) Maximum permissible dose

D) Effective dose

191. Personnel Protection (ALARA)

Question 191:

Which type of shielding material is most effective for X-rays?

A) Aluminum

B) Lead

C) Plastic

D) Rubber

Section 3: The Image Production

192. Image Acquisition and Technical Evaluation

Question 192:

Which image artifact can result from patient motion?

A) Fuzziness

B) Overexposure

C) Underexposure

D) Ghosting

193. Equipment Operation and Quality Assurance

Question 193:

What is the purpose of quality control tests in radiography?

A) To train staff

B) To assess patient satisfaction

C) To validate equipment functionality

D) To reduce costs

Section 4: The Procedures

194. Head, Spine, and Pelvis Procedures

Question 194:

What is the first step in performing a lumbar puncture?

A) Applying local anesthesia

B) Taking a preliminary X-ray

C) Positioning the patient

D) Administering sedation

195. Thorax and Abdomen Procedures

Question 195:

Which view is used to best visualize the diaphragm in chest radiography?

A) AP view

B) PA view

C) Lateral view

D) Oblique view

196. Extremity Procedures

Question 196:

Which bone is commonly fractured in falls involving outstretched hands?

A) Ulna

B) Radius

C) Humerus

D) Scapula

Additional Questions:

197. Ethical and Legal Aspects

Question 197:

Which of the following ethical principles emphasizes "doing no harm" to patients?

A) Autonomy

B) Beneficence

C) Nonmaleficence

D) Justice

198. Principles of Radiation Physics

Question 198:

Which of the following is not a property of X-rays?

A) They are invisible

B) They can be deflected by a magnet

C) They can penetrate opaque materials

D) They can ionize matter

199. Image Acquisition and Technical Evaluation

Question 199:

Which of the following factors primarily affects the contrast of a radiographic image?

A) mA (milliampere)

B) kVp (kilovolt peak)

C) Exposure time

D) Focal length

200. Head, Spine, and Pelvis Procedures

Question 200:

For a head CT scan, which plane is primarily used?

A) Coronal

B) Sagittal

C) Axial

D) Oblique

6.2 Answer Sheet – Practice Test 2

101. Answer:

B) Nonmaleficence

Explanation:

Nonmaleficence means "do no harm" and requires that healthcare professionals avoid harming the patient and actively prevent harm.

102. Answer:

B) Use simple language and props

Explanation:

Using simple language and props helps to make the child comfortable and more cooperative during the procedure.

103. Answer:

C) ECG

Explanation:

An ECG (Electrocardiogram) monitors a patient's heart rate and rhythm.

104. Answer:

B) Lay them flat and elevate the legs

Explanation:

Laying the patient flat and elevating the legs helps to improve blood flow to the brain.

105. Answer:

B) Autoclaving

Explanation:

Autoclaving uses steam under pressure for sterilization.

106. Answer:

D) In a sharps container

Explanation:

Used sharps should be disposed of in a sharps container to prevent needlestick injuries.

107. Answer:

B) Sedative

Explanation:

Sedatives are often used to relax patients before procedures like an MRI.

108. Answer:

C) Electron

Explanation:

In beta decay, an electron is ejected from the nucleus.

109. Answer:

C) Sensitivity to radiation

Explanation:

Radiosensitive means that a tissue or cell is more susceptible to the harmful effects of radiation.

110. Answer:

D) Magnification

Explanation:

The cardinal rules of radiation protection are Time, Distance, and Shielding. Magnification is not one of them.

111. Answer:

A) As Low As Reasonably Achievable

Explanation:

ALARA stands for "As Low As Reasonably Achievable," emphasizing the need to minimize radiation exposure.

112. Answer:

B) Tube voltage

Explanation:

Tube voltage (kVp) primarily affects the contrast of an X-ray image.

113. Answer:

B) Beam alignment test

Explanation:

The beam alignment test ensures that the X-ray beam is properly aligned with the image receptor.

114. Answer:

C) Lateral

Explanation:

The lateral projection is often used to visualize the cervical spine.

115. Answer:

A) 1/60 second

Explanation:

The standard exposure time for a chest X-ray is typically 1/60 second to minimize motion blur.

116. Answer:

B) Oblique

Explanation:

An oblique view of the hand is typically used to visualize a Bennett's fracture.

117. Answer:

A) Battery

Explanation:

Battery in radiology refers to touching the patient without informed consent, which is an intentional tort.

118. Answer:

D) Paraphrasing and asking clarifying questions

Explanation:

Active listening involves paraphrasing the speaker's words and asking clarifying questions for a better understanding.

119. Answer:

B) Blood pressure

Explanation:

Blood pressure is usually the last vital sign to change in a deteriorating patient and is a late indicator of distress.

120. Answer:

B) Rescue, Alarm, Contain, Extinguish

Explanation:

RACE stands for Rescue, Alarm, Contain, and Extinguish, which are the steps to follow in the event of a fire.

121. Answer:

C) 60%

Explanation:

An effective hand sanitizer should contain at least 60% alcohol to be effective against most types of germs.

122. Answer:

A) Daily

Explanation:

Eyewash stations should be checked daily to ensure they are functioning properly and are accessible.

123. Answer:

B) Naloxone

Explanation:

Naloxone is used as a reversal agent for an opioid overdose and can quickly restore normal breathing.

124. Answer:

C) Photoelectric effect

Explanation:

In the photoelectric effect, a K-shell electron is ejected when an incoming X-ray photon is absorbed.

125. Answer:

C) Gray

Explanation:

The Gray (Gy) is the SI unit for measuring absorbed dose of ionizing radiation.

126. Answer:

D) Use a higher speed image receptor

Explanation:

Using a higher-speed image receptor can minimize motion blur by reducing the required exposure time.

127. Answer:

B) 50 mSv

Explanation:

The annual dose limit for radiation workers is 50 mSv (5 rem) according to most guidelines.

128. Answer:

C) Pixel size

Explanation:

Spatial resolution is determined by the pixel size; smaller pixels provide higher resolution.

129. Answer:

A) To focus the X-ray beam

Explanation:

The primary purpose of a collimator is to focus and limit the X-ray beam to the area of interest.

130. Answer:

D) Tangential

Explanation:

Tangential views are often used to best visualize skull sutures.

131. Answer:

B) MRI

Explanation:

MRI is most effective for imaging soft tissue due to its high contrast resolution.

132. Answer:

D) Ulnar deviation

Explanation:

The ulnar deviation view is recommended for suspected scaphoid fractures as it provides the best visualization of the scaphoid bone.

133. Answer:

C) Written agreement to treatment after understanding risks and benefits

Explanation:

Informed consent involves the patient's written agreement to proceed with treatment after fully understanding the risks and benefits.

134. Answer:

B) Nodding

Explanation:

Nodding is a form of non-verbal communication that can indicate agreement or understanding.

135. Answer:

C) Neurological status

Explanation:

The Glasgow Coma Scale is used to assess a patient's neurological status based on their verbal, motor, and eye-opening responses.

136. Answer:

C) Call 911

Explanation:

Immediate medical attention is crucial for a stroke. The first action should be to call 911.

137. Answer:

B) Autoclave

Explanation:

Autoclaving is the most effective method for sterilizing surgical instruments as it uses pressurized steam.

138. Answer:

C) Red

Explanation:

Red color coding is universally used for biohazard waste to indicate the risk of infection.

139. Answer:

A) Nitroglycerin

Explanation:

Nitroglycerin is commonly used as a vasodilator to expand blood vessels and improve blood flow.

140. Answer:

A) Increases

Explanation:

Increasing kVp typically increases the penetrating power of the X-ray beam, which improves image quality.

141. Answer:

C) Genetic mutations

Explanation:

Ionizing radiation can cause genetic mutations in human tissue, potentially leading to cancers or other diseases.

142. Answer:

B) Increasing distance from the source

Explanation:

Increasing the distance from the source of radiation is effective in minimizing scatter, according to the inverse square law.

143. Answer:

B) As Low As Reasonably Achievable

Explanation:

ALARA stands for As Low As Reasonably Achievable, emphasizing the need to minimize radiation exposure.

144. Answer:

B) Blurring

Explanation:

Blurring is a common artifact caused by patient motion during image acquisition.

145. Answer:

A) Light field test

Explanation:

A light field test ensures that the X-ray beam and light field are properly aligned.

146. Answer:

A) AP pelvic X-ray

Explanation:

The AP (Anteroposterior) pelvic X-ray is the standard initial imaging study for suspected pelvic fractures.

147. Answer:

B) PET scan

Explanation:

A PET scan is generally the modality of choice for staging lung cancer due to its ability to visualize metabolic activity.

148. Answer:

D) Sesamoid

Explanation:

The sesamoid view is preferred for imaging the first metatarsophalangeal joint as it provides the best visualization of the area.

149. Answer:

B) Guardian

Explanation:

A legal guardian is authorized to sign consent forms for medical procedures involving a minor.

150. Answer:

C) Encourage detailed answers

Explanation:

Open-ended questions facilitate more detailed responses, helping to gather comprehensive information from the patient.

151. Answer:

B) Rapid breathing

Explanation:

Tachypnea refers to rapid breathing, often a sign of respiratory distress or other medical conditions.

152. Answer:

C) N-acetylcysteine

Explanation:

N-acetylcysteine is used as an antidote for acetaminophen (Tylenol) poisoning to prevent liver damage.

153. Answer:

B) Airborne

Explanation:

Airborne isolation is used for patients with tuberculosis to prevent the spread of the airborne bacteria.

154. Answer:

C) Class C

Explanation:

Class C fire extinguishers are designed for electrical fires and are safe to use around electrical equipment.

155. Answer:

A) Warfarin

Explanation:

Warfarin is an anticoagulant that helps prevent and treat blood clots.

156. Answer:

A) Milli-Ampere second

Explanation:

mAs stands for Milli-Ampere second, a unit that quantifies the total X-ray exposure.

157. Answer:

D) Microwave

Explanation:

Microwave radiation is non-ionizing and does not have enough energy to remove tightly bound electrons from atoms.

158. Answer:

C) Shorter exposure time

Explanation:

A shorter exposure time reduces the chance of motion artifacts as it minimizes the time for potential patient movement.

159. Answer:

B) Lead

Explanation:

Lead is commonly used for shielding against X-rays due to its high atomic number and density.

160. Answer:

B) Brightness distribution

Explanation:

A histogram in digital imaging represents the distribution of pixel brightness in the acquired image.

161. Answer:

B) To restrict the X-ray beam

Explanation:

A collimator restricts the X-ray beam size to limit patient exposure and improve image quality.

162. Answer:

C) MRI

Explanation:

MRI is generally contraindicated for patients with pacemakers due to the magnetic fields involved.

163. Answer:

B) Examine the lower gastrointestinal tract

Explanation:

A barium enema is primarily used to examine the lower gastrointestinal tract, including the colon and rectum.

164. Answer:

B) Supination

Explanation:

Supination is recommended for obtaining a lateral wrist radiograph, as it provides optimal visualization.

165. Answer:

C) The right to refuse treatment

Explanation:

The principle of autonomy emphasizes the patient's right to make their own decisions, including the right to refuse treatment.

166. Answer:

B) Crossed arms

Explanation:

Crossed arms can indicate a defensive or anxious posture and may signal that a patient is anxious or uncomfortable.

167. Answer:

C) Pulse oximeter

Explanation:

A pulse oximeter is used to measure blood oxygen saturation, providing valuable data on a patient's respiratory status.

168. Answer:

B) Difficulty breathing

Explanation:

Difficulty breathing is a severe symptom of anaphylaxis, which requires immediate medical attention.

169. Answer:

B) Autoclaving

Explanation:

Autoclaving is the most effective method for sterilization, as it uses high pressure and temperature to kill all forms of microbes.

170. Answer:

B) Sharps container

Explanation:

Sharps should be disposed of in a designated sharps container to prevent injury and cross-contamination.

171. Answer:

B) Dehydration

Explanation:

The main side effect of diuretics is dehydration, as they promote fluid loss through urination.

172. Answer:

B) Sievert

Explanation:

The unit for dose equivalent in radiation exposure is the Sievert, which takes into account the type of radiation and its biological effect.

173. Answer:

D) Blood cells

Explanation:

Blood cells are most sensitive to radiation, as they divide quickly and are more susceptible to DNA damage.

174. Answer:

C) Exposure area

Explanation:

Collimation primarily affects the exposure area by limiting the X-ray beam, thereby reducing patient exposure.

175. Answer:

C) As Low As Reasonably Achievable

Explanation:

ALARA stands for "As Low As Reasonably Achievable," a principle aimed at minimizing radiation exposure.

176. Answer:

C) Focal spot size

Explanation:

Focal spot size directly affects the sharpness of the image; smaller focal spot sizes result in sharper images.

177. Answer:

C) To validate equipment functionality

Explanation:

Quality control tests are performed to validate the functionality and performance of radiographic equipment, ensuring consistent and high-quality images.

178. Answer:

C) Positioning the patient

Explanation:

The first step in performing a lumbar puncture is positioning the patient, usually in a lateral recumbent position, to access the lumbar region properly.

179. Answer:

B) PA view

Explanation:

The PA (posteroanterior) view is most effective for visualizing the diaphragm in chest radiography, offering a less distorted image.

180. Answer:

B) Radius

Explanation:

The radius is the bone most commonly fractured in falls involving an outstretched hand, often referred to as a "Colles' fracture."

181. Answer:

C) A patient understands the risks, benefits, and alternatives

Explanation:

Informed consent means that the patient has been made aware of the risks, benefits, and alternatives to a proposed treatment and has agreed to proceed.

182. Answer:

B) Gaining rapport with the patient

Explanation:

Active listening helps to build rapport and trust with the patient, making them more likely to be forthcoming with information and follow treatment plans.

183. Answer:

B) ECG monitor

Explanation:

An ECG (Electrocardiogram) monitor is used to continuously track heart rate and rhythm.

184. Answer:

D) Standing behind the patient

Explanation:

The first step in the Heimlich maneuver is to stand behind the patient to apply abdominal thrusts effectively.

185. Answer:

C) Alcohol wipes

Explanation:

Alcohol wipes are generally not effective for sterilization; they are more commonly used for disinfection.

186. Answer:

B) Red

Explanation:

A red color-coded bin is generally used for disposing of biohazardous waste.

187. Answer:

C) Analgesics

Explanation:

Analgesics are commonly used for pain relief and include medications like acetaminophen and ibuprofen.

188. Answer:

C) Gamma

Explanation:

Gamma radiation is the most harmful to human tissues as it can penetrate most materials and can cause severe cellular damage.

189. Answer:

D) M

Explanation:

The M (mitotic) phase is the most sensitive to radiation because the cell is dividing and its DNA is most vulnerable at this stage.

190. Answer:

B) Threshold dose

Explanation:

The threshold dose refers to the radiation level below which no harmful or deterministic effects are expected to occur.

191. Answer:

B) Lead

Explanation:

Lead is the most effective shielding material for X-rays due to its high atomic number, which increases its attenuation ability.

192. Answer:

A) Fuzziness

Explanation:

Fuzziness or blurriness can result from patient motion, affecting the clarity and detail of the image.

193. Answer:

C) To validate equipment functionality

Explanation:

Quality control tests are performed to validate the functionality and performance of radiographic equipment, ensuring consistent and high-quality images.

194. Answer:

C) Positioning the patient

Explanation:

The first step in performing a lumbar puncture is positioning the patient, usually in a lateral recumbent position, to access the lumbar region properly.

195. Answer:

B) PA view

Explanation:

The PA (posteroanterior) view is most effective for visualizing the diaphragm in chest radiography, offering a less distorted image.

196. Answer:

B) Radius

Explanation:

The radius is the bone most commonly fractured in falls involving an outstretched hand, often referred to as a "Colles' fracture."

197. Answer:

C) Nonmaleficence

Explanation:

Nonmaleficence is an ethical principle that emphasizes avoiding harm or injury to patients. It is often summarized as "first, do no harm."

198. Answer:

B) They can be deflected by a magnet

Explanation:

X-rays are electromagnetic waves and do not carry a charge. Therefore, they are not deflected by a magnet.

199. Answer:

B) kVp (kilovolt peak)

Explanation:

The kilovolt peak (kVp) primarily affects the contrast of a radiographic image. Higher kVp results in lower contrast and vice versa.

200. Answer:

C) Axial

Explanation:

The axial plane is primarily used for head CT scans, allowing for detailed cross-sectional images.

TEST-TAKING STRATEGIES

As you approach the Radiography Exam, mastering effective test-taking strategies is essential. Additionally, conquering test anxiety ensures you can showcase your true knowledge and skills. Here's a guide to help you navigate the exam confidently:

Test-Taking Strategies: Radiography Exam Mastery

1. **Read the Instructions Thoroughly:**

- Before diving into the questions, carefully read the instructions for each section. Understanding the format and expectations is crucial for efficient navigation.

2. **Time Management:**

- Allocate time wisely for each section. If a question is particularly challenging, mark it and move on. Return to it later if time permits.

3. **Answer Every Question:**

- There's no penalty for guessing, so ensure you provide an answer for every question. If unsure, make an educated guess based on your knowledge.

4. **Prioritize Questions:**

○ Start with questions you find most comfortable. This builds confidence and allows you to accumulate points early in the exam.

5. **Flag and Review:**

○ Flag questions that you find challenging or want to revisit. Use any remaining time at the end to review flagged questions and make adjustments if needed.

6. **Stay Calm and Focused:**

○ Maintain composure, especially if faced with challenging questions. Take a deep breath, focus on the task at hand, and approach each question methodically.

Overcoming Test Anxiety: Strategies for Success

1. **Practice Mindfulness:**

○ Incorporate mindfulness techniques into your study routine. Techniques such as deep breathing and meditation can help manage stress and anxiety.

2. **Simulate Exam Conditions:**

○ During practice tests, recreate exam conditions as closely as possible. Familiarity with the exam environment reduces anxiety on the actual test day.

3. **Positive Visualization:**

○ Visualize success. Imagine yourself confidently answering questions and completing the exam. Positive visualization can boost confidence and reduce anxiety.

4. Healthy Lifestyle Choices:

- Maintain a healthy lifestyle leading up to the exam. Prioritize sleep, stay hydrated, and engage in regular physical activity. A healthy body supports a healthy mind.

5. Break Tasks Into Smaller Steps:

- Break down the exam into smaller, manageable tasks. Focus on one question at a time, preventing overwhelming feelings.

6. Seek Support:

- Talk to peers, mentors, or professionals who have successfully navigated similar exams. Their insights and experiences can offer valuable perspectives and reassurance.

7. Review and Reflect:

- After completing practice tests, reflect on your performance and identify areas for improvement. Addressing weaknesses boosts confidence and reduces anxiety.

By incorporating these test-taking strategies and anxiety management techniques into your preparation, you'll not only excel in the Radiography Exam but also develop skills that serve you well in future academic and professional endeavors.

ADDITIONAL RESOURCES

To enhance your preparation for the Radiography Exam, we have curated a list of additional resources that complement the content provided in this study guide. These resources offer diverse perspectives, practice opportunities, and in-depth coverage to ensure a comprehensive understanding of radiography principles.

Recommended Online Resources:

1. **RadiologyInfo.org:**

- RadiologyInfo.org serves as a valuable online resource providing patient-friendly information about radiologic procedures and therapies. Explore their comprehensive guides and FAQs to deepen your knowledge.

2. **ARRT Online Exam Handbook:**

- The ARRT Online Exam Handbook offers insights into the online exam format, technical requirements, and guidelines. Familiarize yourself with the platform to optimize your exam-day experience.

3. **Radiology Masterclass:**

- Radiology Masterclass provides a range of tutorials, quizzes, and case-based learning to reinforce radiography concepts. Access their extensive library for interactive learning experiences.

4. **Radiopaedia:**

  ○ Radiopaedia is an online collaborative radiology resource. Explore their articles, cases, and quizzes to expand your knowledge and exposure to diverse radiographic scenarios.

5. **Radiologic Technology Journals:**

  ○ Stay updated with the latest research and advancements in radiologic technology by exploring reputable journals such as the "Journal of Medical Imaging and Radiation Sciences."

Recommended Academic Materials:

1. **"Bontrager's Textbook of Radiographic Positioning and Related Anatomy" by John Lampignano and Leslie E. Kendrick:**

  ○ This textbook provides a comprehensive guide to radiographic positioning, helping you master the practical aspects of image acquisition.

2. **"Merrill's Atlas of Radiographic Positioning and Procedures" by Eugene D. Frank and Bruce W. Long:**

  ○ Explore this atlas for detailed illustrations and step-by-step instructions on radiographic positioning techniques, complementing the content covered in the guide.

3. **"Radiologic Science for Technologists" by Stewart C. Bushong:**

  ○ Bushong's textbook offers a solid foundation in radiologic science, covering essential concepts that align with the Radiography Exam's scope.

4. "Review of Radiologic Physics" by Walter Huda:

- Delve into the principles of radiologic physics with this comprehensive review, ensuring a strong understanding of the theoretical aspects tested in the exam.

5. "Radiography Essentials for Limited Practice" by Bruce W. Long and Eugene D. Frank:

- Tailored for those in limited radiography practice, this resource provides focused content on essential topics relevant to the exam.

By exploring these recommended online resources and academic materials, you'll enrich your study experience and deepen your understanding of radiography, setting the stage for success in the Radiography Exam and beyond.

FINAL WORDS

EMBRACE THE RADIOGRAPHIC JOURNEY

As you conclude your journey through the pages of the Radiography Prep Study Guide 2024-2025, remember that you're not just preparing for an exam; you're stepping into a world of possibilities and contributions to healthcare.

Radiography is not just about capturing images; it's about capturing moments that matter. Each X-ray you take has the potential to unveil answers, guide treatments, and make a difference in someone's life. Your journey is not just about passing a test; it's about becoming a vital part of a profession that combines science, technology, and compassion.

Embrace the Challenges:

The path you've chosen is noble but challenging. Embrace the challenges as opportunities to learn and grow. Every question you encounter, every concept you master, brings you closer to becoming a skilled and compassionate radiologic technologist.

You are More Than a Score:

While the Radiography Exam is a milestone, remember that you are more than a test score. You are a future healthcare professional, ready to contribute to patient care, diagnostic accuracy, and the advancement of medical science. Your journey is about making a lasting impact beyond the confines of an examination room.

Persist Through Perseverance:

Persistence is your greatest ally. In moments of doubt, remember the hours you've invested, the challenges you've overcome, and the knowledge you've gained. Persevere through the uncertainties, for success often lies on the other side of persistence.

Radiate Confidence:

As you step into the exam room, radiate confidence. You've equipped yourself with knowledge, honed your skills, and embraced the journey. Trust in your abilities, approach each question with a clear mind, and let your confidence shine through.

Your Future Awaits:

Beyond the exam, a fulfilling career in radiography awaits you. You'll be at the forefront of medical innovation, contributing to diagnoses, treatments, and advancements in healthcare. Your journey doesn't end with the exam; it transforms into a career filled with purpose and continuous learning.

You Are the Future of Radiography:

You are not just a student preparing for an exam; you are the future of radiography. The impact you make will extend far beyond the confines of a classroom. Embrace the responsibility, the challenges, and the opportunities that come with being a part of this dynamic field.

In closing, as you embark on your journey into the world of radiography, carry with you the knowledge, resilience, and passion that brought you here. Your commitment to excellence will not only shape your success in the exam but will also leave a lasting imprint on the future of healthcare.

Best of luck, future radiologic technologists. Your journey is extraordinary, and your potential is boundless.

EXPLORE OUR RANGE OF STUDY GUIDES

At Test Treasure Publication, we understand that academic success requires more than just raw intelligence or tireless effort—it requires targeted preparation. That's why we offer an extensive range of study guides, meticulously designed to help you excel in various exams across the USA.

Our Offerings

- **Medical Exams:** Conquer the MCAT, USMLE, and more with our comprehensive study guides, complete with practice questions and diagnostic tests.

- **Law Exams:** Get a leg up on the LSAT and bar exams with our tailored resources, offering theoretical insights and practical exercises.

- **Business and Management Tests:** Ace the GMAT and other business exams with our incisive guides, equipped with real-world examples and scenarios.

- **Engineering & Technical Exams:** Prep for the FE, PE, and other technical exams with our specialized guides, which delve into both fundamentals and complexities.

- **High School Exams:** Be it the SAT, ACT, or AP tests, our high school range is designed to give you a competitive edge.

- **State-Specific Exams:** Tailored resources to help you with exams unique to specific states, whether it's teacher qualification exams or state civil service exams.

Why Choose Test Treasure Publication?

- **Comprehensive Coverage:** Each guide covers all essential topics in detail.

- **Quality Material:** Crafted by experts in each field.

- **Interactive Tools:** Flashcards, online quizzes, and downloadable resources to complement your study.

- **Customizable Learning:** Personalize your prep journey by focusing on areas where you need the most help.

- **Community Support:** Access to online forums where you can discuss concerns, seek guidance, and share success stories.

Contact Us

For inquiries about our study guides, or to provide feedback, please email us at support@testtreasure.com.

Order Now

Ready to elevate your preparation to the next level? Visit our website www.testtreasure.com to browse our complete range of study guides and make your purchase.

Made in the USA
Monee, IL
14 November 2024

70084817R00092